THE GOATKEEPER'S
VETERINARY BOOK

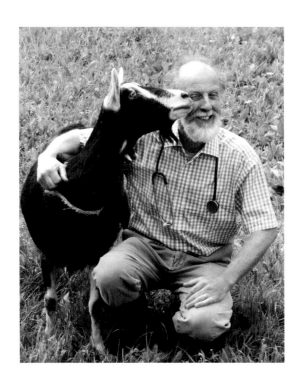

THE GOATKEEPER'S VETERINARY BOOK

Peter Dunn BVSc, MRCVS

ILLUSTRATIONS BY LOUISE DUNN

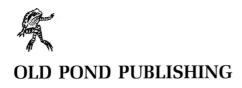

OLD POND PUBLISHING

Cover design by Liz Whatling
Typeset by Galleon Typesetting, Ipswich
Printed and bound in China for Compass Press Limited

CONTENTS

Poisoning
*Lead • fluoride • pentachlorophenol • diesel
fuel • nitrate (nitrite)*

Plant poisoning
*Rhododendron • ragwort • kale • oxalate • oak
leaf • fruit tree leaf*

PREFACE TO THE FOURTH EDITION

The world population of goats is 450 million and their products feed and clothe a substantial number of the human population. Despite this, there is relatively little scientific information available on goats compared to other farmed species. This is because they are generally less important in the agriculture of developed countries, where most of the scientific information is generated. Moving to France has helped me to tap into goat information, in a country where they are an important agricultural species.

It is against this background that I have tried to sift information on goats and present it to the goatkeeper in a readily useable form. The book is intended to be a first point of reference on goat health and disease for the goatkeeper. Seek further advice and clarification from your vet. I hope that you find the book useful and that it adds to your enjoyment of keeping goats.

There is a problem for goatkeepers and veterinarians when it comes to the use of veterinary medicines. The licensing of these medicines is a complex and costly process. It is there to protect the animal and the consumer. There are few licensed products for goats in developed countries because of the poor financial return for the manufacturers. To illustrate this, there are only eleven licensed products for UK goats in the 2004 compendium of data sheets, compared with over 160 for sheep. Sometimes a medicine is licensed for goats in another country and I have tried to indicate this in the text.

If an unlicensed product is used on goats then the 'standard' withdrawal period of seven days should be used before the milk is consumed and twenty-eight days before the meat is consumed by humans. If the withdrawal period for the licensed species is longer than this, then that longer period would apply.

Finally, if any goatkeeper were to ask me for three important tips on goatkeeping, they would be: (1) keep a closed herd, (2) ensure kids receive adequate colostrum, and (3) always include oral electrolytes in the treatment of sick animals. If you haven't got any (commercial) electrolytes to hand, then try a teaspoonful of table salt and a dessertspoonful of glucose dissolved in a litre of warm water.

I am grateful to the following people for their help with various aspects of the photography:

Dr A H Andrews RVC, London University
Jim Berryman, Pardons Cottage, Woods Corner, Dallington, Heathfield, East Sussex TN21 9JX (Back cover)
Dr Alex Donaldson and Jennifer Ryder IVRI, Pirbright
Peter Jackson FRCVS, Cambridge University Veterinary School
David Robins, who very kindly photographed the caesarean sequence

A special thank you to Patricia Wilkinson who took the front cover photograph, despite the old adage about not working with children or animals.

A 'merci' is also in order for Thierry Bazin, our local goat technician for his useful comments and help and also to Christophe Foreix for allowing me to take photographs.

I also wish to thank Dr R J Esselemont, Department of Agriculture, Earley Gate, University of Reading, Reading RG6 2AT, for the Daisy information system example.

Finally, a big thank you to Louise, my wife, for all her hard work looking after our goats and for her encouragement.

PETER DUNN

Chapter 1

PRINCIPLES OF HEALTH AND MANAGEMENT

HEALTH AND DISEASE

The emphasis of this book is on keeping goats healthy and free from disease. The word 'disease' describes precisely what it is: *dis-ease*, the state when an animal is not at ease with its surroundings. Health is more difficult to define but it is the state when an animal is at ease with its surroundings. Common usage has resulted in the word disease being equated with infections, whereas the situation is, in fact, far more complex.

The factors that decide whether or not an animal succumbs to a disease condition are many and varied. They can be conveniently categorised, however, as:

1. The goat's own peculiarities
2. The surroundings in which we keep it
3. The infectious agents in that environment.

All three groups of factors influence each other, as represented in Figure 1.1. One could consider health to be the state of affairs

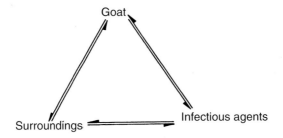

FIGURE 1.1   Factors determining health and disease

when a balance is struck between these three factors. Disease on the other hand occurs when there is an imbalance of these forces.

The Goat's Defence Mechanisms Against Disease

There are three types of defence mechanism:

1. General defence and the normal functioning of the goat
2. Cellular defence system
3. Humoral (antibody) system.

The General Defence System

Examples of the general defence system are the skin, which covers the body and protects it from invasion; the acidity of the true stomach, which destroys some micro-organisms taken in with the food; and also the upper respiratory tract. The latter contains the turbinate bones in the nose which trap particles of dust before they enter the air passages. This function is assisted by the mucus lining the whole of the air-conducting part of the system.

The Cellular Defence System

Special cells (microphages and macrophages) found in the tissues and circulating bloodstream are capable of destroying micro-organisms that have entered the goat's body. They accomplish this by phagocytosis, literally eating up and digesting the invader.

The Humoral (Antibody) Defence System

Specific antibodies capable of inactivating bacteria and viruses are found in abundance in the goat's tissues. Antibody is also produced against worm parasites but it is generally fairly poor and short-lived. The production of antibody always follows exposure to a specific micro-organism. Repeated exposure increases the quantity produced. The process is mimicked in vaccination when minute doses of inactivated micro-organism (or part of the micro-organism) are given to the goat to stimulate its production of antibody. Commonly used vaccines for goats are against tetanus and enterotoxaemia.

Susceptibility and Resistance

All goats are either susceptible or resistant to diseases with all the grades in between. When considering infectious diseases, the key to avoiding problems is to know which goats are susceptible and which are immune. Kids are susceptible to most diseases because they have not developed antibody against them. If they have received adequate colostrum, however, they are protected against most of the diseases to which the dam is immune. This maternal immunity rapidly declines over the first few weeks of life and the kid must then start to manufacture its own antibodies.

Colostrum is the first milk produced by the newly kidded mother. In the case of goats, no antibodies pass directly from dam to kid in the uterus. The antibodies pass to the kid in the colostrum.

Gradual exposure to most disease agents can be considered to be akin to a natural vaccination process. Goatkeepers must be aware that a kid's resistance may be very different from an adult's, and they must plan accordingly. It would be unwise, for example, to mix a large group of adult goats in the same house as a large group of kids. The kids would be very prone to respiratory disease. Similarly when at pasture the kid is very much more susceptible to worm parasites than its dam.

Stress and Disease

The word 'stress' is frequently used in this modern age to refer to the 'stress' of business life or of living in a big city. We all think we know what stress is, but when does it become involved in goat disease? One famous biologist (Seleye) put forward a theory to explain the exact mechanism of stress. His view was that any detrimental influence on an animal, such as a goat, is a stressor. These influences are legion and diverse, but include factors such as bullying by other goats, overcrowding, long journeys and climatic factors such as heat. The crux of the matter is that they are all transmitted by the goat's brain, and have a common effect on the physiology (or internal workings) of the goat. This effect is thought to be the release of excessive quantities of hormone from the adrenal cortex. The adrenalin hormone is released from the medulla of the gland and (coincidentally) corticosteroid hormones are released from the adrenal cortex (the outer part of the gland). Hormones are 'chemical messengers', that are released into the bloodstream. These corticosteroid hormones reduce the goat's defence mechanisms and therefore render it more susceptible to infectious diseases (*see* Figure 1.2).

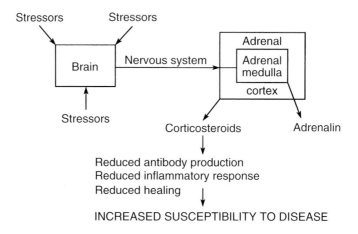

FIGURE 1.2   Stress and disease

GOOD STOCKMANSHIP

Everyday dealings with goats, or other animals for that matter, should be directed to reducing stress, which means simply that common sense in feeding, housing and management are needed. For example, avoid sudden changes in diet and avoid unsuitable floors that lead to goats slipping and injuring themselves. It is all the little points that distinguish good goatkeepers from bad ones, and this manifests itself in the health of their animals.

The Importance of Good Husbandry
Over the last decade research work on the dairy cow has shown that poor husbandry is the most important factor in numerous common disease conditions such as mastitis, acetonaemia, infertility and lameness. All these points are equally applicable to goat husbandry, and remember that avoiding disease by good husbandry saves money on veterinary fees.

Preventive Medicine

Obviously, the aim of all goatkeepers is to promote good health and avoid disease in their animals. Using vaccines, worm preparations and suchlike are some of the ways of achieving this goal. Disease can be prevented, of course, by practising the best kind of husbandry, and advice can be obtained on this. Some goatkeepers with large herds arrange a regular visit by their veterinary surgeon in order to discuss this very point. Such a visit is aimed at going over the routines of the farm and identifying areas where advice is needed. It may be, for example, that a ten-minute discussion on mastitis control can save you milk that would otherwise have been lost through this costly disease.

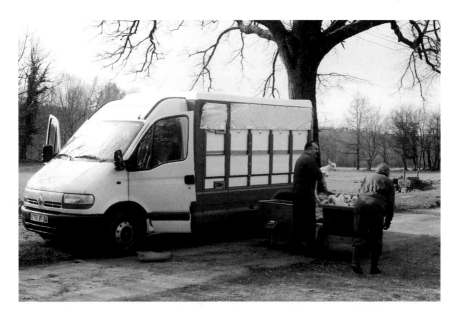

PLATE 1.1   Biosecurity. Keep livestock carriers and their drivers away from your stock. Take stock for collection to the perimeter of your property.

Herd Health Plans

For many farm species, modern farmers compile a health plan with their vet. This sets out the farms policy and action plan for many aspects of animal husbandry. This is a method of focussing on prevention and planning to avoid problems as well as knowing what action would be taken should they arise.

Using the example of mastitis, the plan would consider the past problems, recommendations would be listed and perhaps targets agreed. A standard operating plan would be discussed. This would list the action to be taken through the year, for example, a check of the milking machine in January.

Guidelines of how to treat clinical cases of mastitis would be agreed. For example, the herdsman would be given a list of things to do, so that action could be taken immediately without having to discuss the matter with the vet whilst in the middle of milking.

This might be a list such as:

- Hold the goat back until the others have been milked.
- Mark her on the back using a red crayon.
- Using a sample tube supplied by the vet, collect a clean sample after the initial teat disinfection, discarding the first few squirts into a receptacle.
- Milk the goat, discarding the milk into a bucket or pour on the muck heap.
- Insert a syringe of vet-supplied antibiotic.
- Teat-dip the goat.
- Take the rectal temperature of the goat.
- Write down the goat's number on the blackboard (Especially if a different milker may be involved). Make a note to contact the vet the next day.
- Place a coloured tape around the goat's leg, on the affected side.
- Place the labelled sample in the fridge bearing the goats number.
- Record the details in the medicines book.
- Increase the supply of straw by 20 per cent to improve the hygiene of the bedding.
- Contact your vet to discuss whether to send off the sample for laboratory investigation.

Similar routines would be planned for lame goats, diarrhoea cases and suchlike. The routines of young kids would then be methodically considered in order to identify treatment, procedures and possibly vaccination plans. A similar plan should be made for rearing stock.

VACCINES AND VACCINATION

Vaccines are an economical method of protecting goats against some diseases. Used in accordance with the manufacturer's instructions they are normally safe and effective. They are not magic potions and, for example, the goats must be adequately fed if they are to be able to respond to them. Likewise, the ability of a goat to defend itself wanes as old age approaches.

Some vaccines (such as enterotoxaemia vaccine) contain adjuvants. These are compounds such as aluminium hydroxide which enhance the immune response by prolonging the release of vaccine from the injection site. They tend to cause 'lumps' at the site of injection, which may persist for months. Injections are therefore best administered inside the foreleg or at other sites where the lumps are not visible. The following points should be observed when using vaccines.

1. Follow the instructions for use carefully.

2. Check the expiry date in case the vaccine is out of date.

3. Be 'clean' when administering vaccines; Avoid wet coats and cross contamination. When using one (new) needle for each goat, it is not necessary to swab the site with spirit or alcohol. If multi-dose containers are used avoid contaminating the vaccine with a dirty needle. Always use two needles, one in the container and one for injecting the goat. Thus needle A is used to draw the vaccine into the syringe, the syringe is disconnected from needle A and needle B is used for injecting the goat. For the next goat the procedure is repeated so that needle A always remains in the vaccine bottle. Ideally a new needle is used for each goat.

4. Avoid injecting or pricking yourself. This is especially important if using vaccines against orf or toxoplasma.

5. Keep a record of dates when vaccines were given.

6. Check the minimum age of receiving the vaccine; for instance, for enterotoxaemia this is ten weeks for kids born to vaccinated does, one week for kids born to unvaccinated does.

7. Remember CAE (caprine arthritis encephalitis virus) can be transmitted from one goat to another by using the same (unsterile) needle.

Signs of Health and Ill Health

Recognising that goats are sick is easy when something very obvious such as bloat occurs. Being able to spot the more subtle indications of ill health is rewarding because treatment can be initiated quickly. This may mean fewer deaths or fewer animals becoming ill because action is taken in time. The signs that the goatkeeper should monitor every day are listed below:

- *General attitude*: alert, inquisitive
- *Appetite*: the goat should be interested in food at almost any time. Excess thirst is a bad sign
- *Cudding*: at certain times of the day your goat should chew the cud. The goat normally cuds after a period of feeding or grazing, so one should see cudding within a period of 3–4 hours
- *The eyes and nose*: bright eyes, no discharges and a cool, dry nose
- *The coat*: clean and glossy
- *The droppings*: firm and pelleted
- *The urine*: light brown, no blood in it
- *Breathing*: regular and unlaboured
- *The gait*: steady, all feet taking weight as the goat walks
- *Milk yield*: sudden changes should be noted
- *The milk*: changes such as clots or blood are abnormal
- *Reproductive signs*: goats on heat.

BE OBSERVANT: In order to notice deviation from normality one must be very familiar with the normal situation. All goatkeepers should be unconsciously noticing little points about their stock as they tend them. Anything abnormal should be carefully noted in case it turns out to be significant.

Nursing Sick Goats

Goats have a reputation for being poor patients in that they seem to give up the will to live. Therefore, it is all the more important that goatkeepers be diligent in nursing their charges. From observing sick animals on different farms and smallholdings it has become clear to me that some people have a gift for nursing while others do not. The veterinary surgeon can only prescribe and treat sick animals; the owners must carry out the important task of nursing.

Firstly, like humans, animals respond to their surroundings, so put them in a pleasant, airy building, with light and possibly access to the outside. The floor should be well strawed up. Avoid shutting goats up in a north-facing 'Black Hole of Calcutta'. Water should always be on offer, but not food. If a goat is not eating offer it a range of titbits from time to time, but try to avoid leaving uneaten food with the animal for long periods. Offer only small quantities and choose appetising or unusual foodstuffs. For example, a sick goat will often nibble at apple tree prunings or ivy leaves. Once the patient starts to eat, gradually encourage it with increased quantities.

The approach one takes obviously depends upon the condition being nursed. Animals with severe pneumonia, for example, would benefit from having their water supply raised. Never be afraid to let a sick animal outside if it shows any desire to go out. A nibble at greenery may do it the world of good. A dilemma for herd owners when they have one sick goat is whether to turn it out with the rest of the herd. Goats are herd animals and get very upset when kept in alone. This can even delay recovery because they are stressed by the separation. Sometimes a compromise is best. Keep the animal in for long enough to provide the individual treatment required and then let it re-join the herd.

Bed Sores

Goats that are 'down' for long periods soon develop sore patches of skin where they are in contact with bedding. Keep the bedding as dry as possible and reposition the goat twice a day. Encourage it to stand occasionally. Goats should never be allowed to lie flat on their sides for long periods but should be encouraged to sit on their brisket (propped if necessary), to avoid risk of bloat.

The Animal's State of Mind

Some goats that have been 'down' for some days become convinced that they cannot get up. Often they will get up if they are encouraged and if the goatkeeper assists by supporting their rear quarters. With help, try carrying a recumbent goat to a new environment, this sometimes stimulates struggling, resulting in the goat getting up.

General Treatments

Specific treatments have been dealt with in other parts of this book but a few general comments are applicable here. Fluid therapy is increasingly used for many conditions with good results, especially when the goat will not eat. This means that fluids and salts are administered either orally or by injection. Many veterinary surgeons find intravenous injections such as glucose-saline solution or Duphalyte (Fort Dodge) useful in these instances. Many commercial oral rehydration preparations are available, to give a similar effect, such as Lectade (Pfizer limited). These can be easily administered by the owner. I find offering a sick goat the following warm drink very useful. Dissolve one dessertspoonful (50 g) of glucose plus a teaspoonsful (10 g) of table salt in a litre of tepid water.

WHEN TO SEEK HELP FROM THE VET

It is extremely difficult to give any general rules as to when a goatkeeper should seek the help of his or her vet because it depends partly on the goatkeeper's experience. By looking up the relevant section in this book you will hopefully receive some guidance, but that often presupposes that you know what you are dealing with. Most vets are prepared to answer simple questions on the phone, but remember that they do not earn any money during these conversations and they are not getting their calls done.

Seek Attention Quickly in the Following Circumstances:

- Broken limbs
- Severe bleeding
- Goats with nervous symptoms
- Prostrate goats
- Suspected poisoning
- Protracted birth of kids
- Prolapse of the womb after kidding (*see* photo page 209)
- Bloated goats.
- Depressed goats with cold nose and body temperature below 35°C

Delays can be detrimental; give your vet plenty of warning so that in the case of a difficult kidding, for instance, he has a chance to deliver live kids. Seek help less urgently with goats that refuse food for longer than eight hours or for goats with clots in the milk.

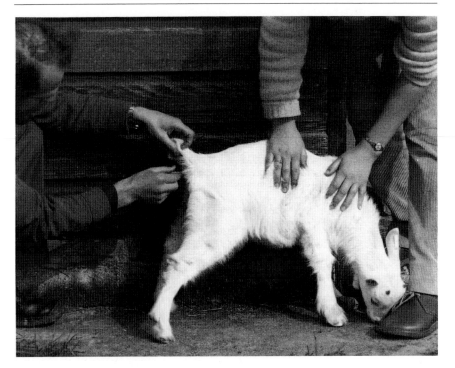

PLATE 1.2   Taking the temperature of a kid

Buying Stock

Your Foundation Goats

A few points should be considered when you are buying your
first goats. If your premises has had no goats on it for over two
years it should be free from most infectious disease problems of
goats. This is a wonderful opportunity to start off with a clean
bill of health. If the ground that you intend to keep your goats on
has carried sheep, then you can be less sure of a clean start
because goats and sheep have many diseases in common.

Examine your prospective purchase carefully, if possible in
daylight. Pay particular attention to:

- Bright eyes
- Alert expression
- Absence of discharge from the eyes and the nose
- A goat that stands well and square; not a goat that keeps
  wanting to lie down. (Is it lame?)

- Look for cud chewing, but avoid a goat that 'drops its cud' or drools saliva (adult)
- Avoid goats that breath excessively fast at rest, or goats with diarrhoea
- Look for a clean healthy-looking coat which is free of parasites
- The udder attachment should be over a large area, with average-length teats (not too long). Feel the udder which should be soft and free from hard lumps (adults). Check that there are only two teats
- Check for other obvious problems such as a hernia, abscesses
- Examine the front teeth in order to assess the goat's age
- Fibre producing goats (Angora) fleece/results of last clip
- In dairy goats, milk production records.

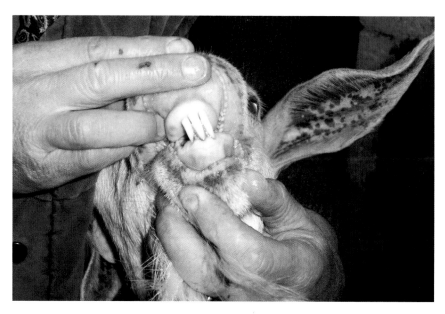

PLATE 1.3   Examine the front teeth – this goat has lost some incisors

General

Enquire from the owner if and when the goat was vaccinated, and obtain the date of the last worm treatment. Ask the vendor if any of their goats have had Johne's disease; if the answer is 'yes' then avoid purchasing goats from that source (*see* JOHNE'S DISEASE, page 133). Find out from the owner how the animal has been kept for the previous six months: whether it has been out at pasture, inside all the time, or whatever. This is especially necessary when purchasing young kids, and you should also be sure to obtain a clear picture of the diet of young kids. Look at any other animals on the premises while you are there and note any signs of ill health that might affect your purchase. You may decide to ask your vet to give your prospective goat a health examination, and it could be arranged that you will return the animal if your vet advises you against buying it. It is advisable to buy goats only from stock which have been tested for CAE (*see* page 226). There should be three clear tests with a six-month interval between them, i.e. one year from the first test to the last one. Demand to see the test results before buying.

When You Get Them Home

Ensure the goats have clean fresh water offered in a receptacle that *cannot* be fouled by droppings. If possible, house them for the first 48 hours, especially if you are going to worm them; this avoids the goats contaminating your new pasture with worm eggs and larvae (*see* Chapter 5.) Offer some hay to goats of all ages, but avoid over-feeding. If the goat is lactating, feed her exactly what the previous owner fed her, but certainly no more. Non-lactating goats are best fed smaller quantities than normal, especially after a long journey. Young kids below six weeks, previously fed with milk or milk replacer, should be offered one feed of electrolyte solution. If this is not available, have their ration halved for the first feed. Then, after an hour, offer tepid water with a teaspoonful (10 g) of table salt per litre. In general you will get few problems if goats are under-fed for the first few days, but many more if they are over-fed. If your goats have not been vaccinated against enterotoxaemia contact your veterinary surgeon to have this done. Consider lice control (*see* page 247), it would be ideal to treat them newly purchased. Ask the vendor for details of all recent treatments.

Herd Management Policy

It is important to consider this before you start your herd. One can either keep a herd which is 'open' to goats coming in to it, or establish a 'closed' herd where one strives to avoid any new goats coming in, once it has been established. The reason, of course, is to reduce the chances of buying in problems. Whenever one buys in stock one buys in different germs at the same time. After a few months of having established a closed herd the foundation goats will have 'swapped' any micro-organisms that they were carrying and all the goats will live in harmony with them. This can be an ideal situation and less disease is likely, compared to an open herd where goats are subsequently bought in. The drawback of the closed herd policy is, of course, in relation to breeding. After some years no new genes are available and the herd can become inbred.

Two methods to get around this are using artificial insemination (AI) or possibly embryo transfer. AI is common in many countries and carries very little risk of infection entering the herd.

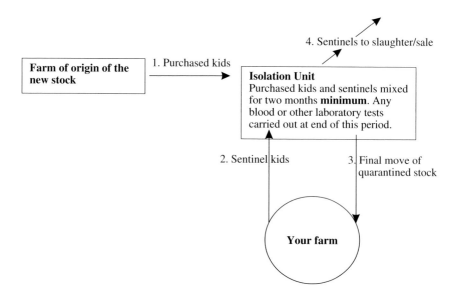

FIGURE 1.3   *A suggested protocol for the buying-in of new bloodlines into a semi-closed herd*

If neither of these options is available then one is forced to break the closed herd policy.

In this case careful selection of sires from a known high-health status herd will reduce any risk. The incoming males can then be isolated from the new herd for a period of perhaps two months. By purchasing young male kids removed from their mothers at 24 hours, one will further reduce the possibility of bringing in problems. Ideally they could be reared at another holding with no livestock but mixed with a few kids of low value from the destination herd (sentinel kids). By this method, any diseases that the new kids may be carrying would show up in these sentinel kids. Thus appropriate action could be taken before admitting them into the destination herd. The sentinel kids are best disposed of to slaughter or sale and not returned to the main herd. (*See* diagram on page 14.)

GOATKEEPERS AND THE LAW

Goatkeepers in the UK are required by law to have a copy of the 'Code of Recommendations for the Welfare of Goats' (PB0081). It is available free from Defra Publications, ADMAIL 6000, London SW1A 2XX, Tel: 0845 955 6000.

Notifiable Diseases (Reportable Diseases USA)

Certain diseases affecting goats are listed as being 'notifiable' by the Department of Environment, Food and Rural Affairs (Defra), or the equivalent government veterinary service in other countries. They tend to be infectious and contagious diseases that affect all ruminants, and in order to control them it is necessary to have co-operation between the owners and the government. By law Defra must be informed if they are suspected. More information can be obtained on the internet on the following pages: http://defraweb.gov.uk/animalh/diseases/notifiable/index.htm.

Contact your local Animal health divisional office of Defra. Your local office can be found from the Defra website: www.defra.gov.uk.

The list of notifiable diseases applicable to goats in the UK is:

- Anthrax
- Bluetongue
- Contagious Agalactia
- Foot-and-mouth Disease
- Peste Des Petits Ruminants
- Rift Valley Fever
- Aujeszky's Disease
- Brucellosis (Melitensis)
- Contagious Epididymitis
- Goat Pox
- Rabies
- Scrapie.

Apart from scrapie, these disease are not present in the UK. I will make a brief summary of each of the notifiable diseases below or refer the reader to where it is covered in more detail in this book.

Anthrax (*see* page 224)

Aujeszky's Disease (*see* page 228)

Bluetongue

This is an insect-borne viral disease to which all species of ruminants are susceptible, although sheep are the most severely affected. Cattle are the main ruminant reservoir of the virus and are very important in the pattern of the disease. It affects the linings of the mouth and nose, and the coronary band of the foot.

The symptoms are varied, ranging from mild to potentially severe, in some cases even resulting in death. Sheep may have a fever and increased respiration. Around the head there may be swelling, inflamed lips, nose and tongue. Excess salivation and nasal discharge may be present. Lameness may be noticed. Following on from this, loss of condition and abortion may occur. Goats are quite resistant to the disease, although some reports describe the symptoms as being similar to those seen in sheep.

Brucellosis (Melitensis) (*see* page 194)

Contagious Agalactia (Agalactia)

This is an infectious mycoplasmal disease of sheep and goats present in many parts of the world. The incubation period can vary from seven days to two months. The symptoms commence with fevered animals (41 to 42°C) some of which may die. As the disease progresses symptoms of arthritis, mastitis and abortion are noted. The nature of the milk becomes yellow. The udder reduces in size (atrophies) and milk yield falls. The eyes can become affected and blindness may result. The joints become swollen and painful. In many countries control is through an eradication policy and the slaughter of affected herds. Vaccines are available for use in countries that do not have a slaughter policy.

Contagious Epidydimitis

This disease of sheep is caused by *Brucella ovis*. It results in a fever in rams which subsequently become infertile, due to the infection localising in the epididymis of the testicles. It is not thought to occur naturally in goats but it can be produced experimentally. Its distribution includes Australia, New Zealand, the USA and parts of Europe.

Foot and Mouth Disease (*see* page 230)

Goat Pox. Capripox (*see also* page 167)
Goat pox is a serious, contagious viral disease of goats. Sheep pox and Goat pox are thought to be caused by the same virus. The virus is spread by the respiratory route and is most likely to occur with crowding and gathering of stock. During outbreaks many goats will become ill and in goats not immune to this virus, mortality may be very high, especially among kids. A trace of this virus in scabs or buildings may be infective for up to six months.

Distribution
It is endemic in most of Africa, the Middle East and Asia.

Symptoms
Initial signs are rapid onset of fever, salivation, nasal discharge and conjunctivitis. Skin lesions erupt within a few days. These develop into vesicles, followed by pustules and scabs. Small red spotty areas appear on the udder and teats, which may burst and form scabs. Affected skin is very sensitive. Internal lesions in the lungs can result in respiratory distress. In resistant animals skin lesions are mild. Death can occur due to the effects of the virus or due to secondary bacterial septicaemia.

Transmission can be through direct contact or contamination from dirty vehicles, housing etc.

There is no treatment. In many countries control is by slaughter of the infected animals.

Vaccination
In many countries attenuated virus vaccines are available, providing immunity for up to two years.

Peste Des Petits Ruminants
The symptoms of this disease in a non-immune sheep and goat population are very severe. It is caused by a virus (morbillivirus) and is similar to rinderpeste. In the acute form the goats are fevered (40–41°C) showing restlessness, dry muzzles, and are off food. Runny nasal discharges later become thickened and then crust over. This blocks the nostrils causing respiratory distress. Concurrently the eyes become reddened and discharges develop. Diarrhoea, coughing and abortion follow, the goats becoming emaciated and dying within five to ten days. The incubation period is short and diseased goats and sheep infect others by

infectious droplets. Spread tends to be through close contact between animals. Goats are generally more severely affected than sheep. In many parts of Africa this is a very serious economic problem of livestock.

Rabies

This unpleasant disease can affect all warm-blooded animals, including humans. Goats would normally become infected through the bite of a dog or fox. The virus affects the nervous system leading to changes in behaviour. The incubation period can be very long between two weeks and six months. Frequently, affected animals salivate excessively and this saliva is infectious to other animals and humans. Even goats may become aggressive and bite, continuous bleating is also reported. The disease is almost always fatal and gradually the stricken animal would become paralysed and die if not euthanased. Rabies is not infrequently recorded in goats in Eastern Europe where the disease is present in the wildlife population.

Control in the UK is by a strict quarantine policy. Imported animals would be the most suspect.

Rift Valley Fever

This is another serious viral disease of ruminants in Africa, which can cause an unpleasant flu-like disease in humans. It affects cattle, sheep, goats and wild ruminants. The disease results in high death rates in young animals and significant numbers of abortions and illness in adult ruminants. It has a short incubation period of one to three days.

It is mainly spread by insects but direct contact can also result in disease, humans become infected from handling infected animals or meat.

Symptoms in sheep and goats include high fever (40–42°C), lack of appetite, weakness and death within 36 hours in young animals. In adults, a thick nasal discharge and vomiting are classic symptoms. Again, recently imported animals would be the most likely suspects.

Scrapie (*see* page 237)

If British goatkeepers suspect these diseases they should contact their veterinary surgeon, or the Divisional Veterinary Manager, Defra (Department for environment, food and rural affairs). Should these diseases be confirmed, Defra has wide-ranging

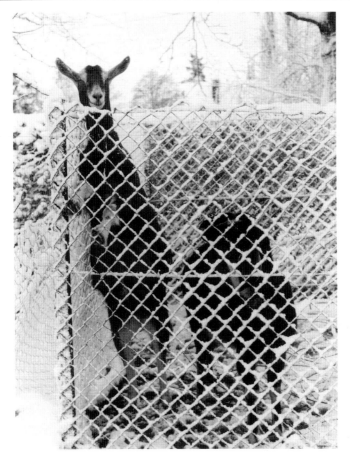

PLATE 1.4   Given shelter goats survive the hardest winter

powers to deal with the situation. Each country has its own list of diseases, and overseas readers should check with their government veterinary service.

Movement Records

In order to be able to trace possible contacts in the event of an outbreak of a notifiable disease, the law stipulates that goat-keepers must keep a record of the movements of their animals. Records should be kept of does being taken to the buck or to shows or any other movements. Movement record books can be obtained from your local authority. An AML1 licence must accompany the goats on the journey.

Production Records and Recording

Many commercial goatkeepers derive great benefit from being members of organisations which process data from their farms and provide the results in an easily understandable format. This

```
HERD :   1 -                                                                    DAISY   B2
NAME                                                                            DATE 18APR94
                                                                                PAGE    1
ADDRESS
...............................................................................................
WEEKLY MANAGEMENT REPORT :  129 MILKING
...............................................................................................

Sorted by calving date
   then cow name
```

	LAC STATUS	Calving Date	Days Open	Num	Date (SERVICE)	Sire	Mas	Lam	NUMBER Days in milk	Peak	MILK YIELD so far	Recordings 29OCT	28NOV	29DEC	CAR	% weekly change	Est. 305d yield	Conc kg per day last	this	Score	GRP
97	2 US /	10JAN90	1559*	0			0	0	1084	5.1	3483	1.8	1.7	1.5		-2.8	1320				1
112	2 US /	14JAN90	1555*	0			0	0	1080	6.1	4185	2.1	2.4	2.5		0.9	1634				1
116	2 US /	22APR90	1457*	0			0	0	982	5.7	3404	2.7	2.7	2.4		-2.6	1296				1
181	2 P+ /	5JAN91	629*	1(2JUL93)WGM40D			0	0	724	4.6	2594	2.1	1.8	1.9		1.2	1241				2
289	1 P+ /	28JUN91	453*	1(30JUN93)WGM40D			0	0	519	3.3	1220	2.2	1.8	0.0		0.0	711				2
290	1 P+ /	6SEP91	382*	1(29JUN93)WGM40D			0	0	449	4.0	1358	0.0	1.9	0.0		0.0	999				2
299	1 US /	19SEP91	942*	0			0	0	467	4.2	1605	2.3	2.9	2.0		-8.2	1114				2
21	4 US /	50CT91	926*	0			0	0	451	4.1*	1430	2.0	1.6	1.7		1.3	1102				2
220	2 US /	50CT91	926*	0			0	0	451	5.1	1721	3.3	2.7	2.4		-2.6	1250				2
120	3 US /	130CT91	918*	0			0	0	443	4.8	1380	2.0	0.5	0.7	CU	7.5	1174				2
133	3 P+ /	140CT91	349*	1(4JUL93)WGM40D			0	0	411	3.3*	1034	1.6	1.1	0.0		0.0	826				2
154	3 US /	170CT91	914*	0			0	0	439	3.9*	1495	2.8	3.2	3.0		-1.4	1084				2
141	5 US /	180CT91	913*	0			0	0	438	3.1*	1084	2.0	2.0	1.5		-6.4	826				2
93	4 US /	1JAN92	838*	0			0	0	363	4.6	1391	2.1	2.6	3.3		5.3	1233				2
32	4 US /	2JAN92	837*	0			0	0	362	4.3*	1069	2.0	1.7	1.2		-7.7	973				1
182	3 US /	2JAN92	837*	0			0	0	362	4.3*	1221	2.4	2.8	2.4		-3.4	1072				2
243	2 US /	2JAN92	837*	0			0	0	362	4.3	1338	3.8	3.8	2.5		-9.3	1140				1
189	3 US /	3JAN92	836*	0			0	0	361	4.3*	1170	2.4	1.9	2.0		1.1	1053				2
155	3 US /	6JAN92	833*	0			0	0	358	4.4*	1299	2.8	4.0	2.1		-14.0	1128				2
194	3 US /	8JAN92	831*	0			0	0	356	4.1*	1005	2.5	1.0	1.4		7.5	932				2
199	3 US /	11JAN92	828*	0			0	0	353	3.9*	1099	2.2	2.1	2.4		3.0	991				1
212	3 US /	11JAN92	828*	0			0	0	353	6.8	1933	4.1	3.7	3.2		-3.2	1758				1
203	3 US /	14JAN92	825*	0			0	0	350	3.6*	1082	2.2	2.4	2.4		0.0	976				1
240	2 US /	15JAN92	824*	0			0	0	349	4.2	1070	3.0	1.7	2.0		3.6	980				1
301	1 US /	17JAN92	822*	0			0	0	347	4.4	1336	3.4	3.6	3.2		-2.6	1193				2
244	2 US /	18JAN92	821*	0			0	0	346	3.8*	1059	2.2	2.1	2.5		3.9	966				1
233	2 US /	20JAN92	819*	0			0	0	344	3.9*	1011	2.2	2.1	2.0		-1.1	928				2
249	2 US /	20JAN92	819*	0			0	0	344	5.0	1258	2.8	2.9	3.2		2.2	1139				1
302	1 US /	23JAN92	816*	0			0	0	341	4.3	1157	2.8	2.6	2.9		2.4	1057				1
144	3 US /	24JAN92	815*	0			0	0	340	4.6	1115	2.0	1.8	2.1		3.4	1045				1
33	3 US /	27JAN92	812*	0			0	0	337	4.0*	940	2.0	2.0	1.3		-9.5	885				2
160	3 US /	27JAN92	812*	0			0	0	337	5.6	1338	3.0	3.5	2.4		-8.4	1242				2
272	2 US /	28JAN92	811*	0			0	0	336	4.6	1124	2.6	2.5	2.4		-0.9	1046				2
94	3 P+ /	30JAN92	300*	1(1SEP93)WGM40D			0	0	334	4.4*	1094	2.0	2.2	1.9		-3.3	1033				2
303	1 US /	30JAN92	809*	0			0	0	334	4.5	1210	3.1	3.2	2.8		-3.0	1123				2

FIGURE 1.4　*Form used in the Daisy Dairy Goat Management System, Department of Agriculture, Reading University, UK*

helps the goatkeeper to keep a check on fertility and production in order to get the best from the herd. An example of the type of print-out supplied is shown on page 20:

THE GOATKEEPER'S VETERINARY CUPBOARD

1 clinical thermometer
1 pair 6-inch scissors,
   round-ended, curved
Sharp knife
Hoof shears
1 pair 15 cm forceps
1 lamb reviver (stomach tube)
A torch
Cotton wool
Several bandages 5 m × 5 cm
Box of adhesive plasters
Soap
50 ml tincture of iodine

Antiseptic/disinfectant such
   as Dettol
Antiseptic powder
Surgical spirit
Vaseline petroleum jelly
Bicarbonate of soda
1 tin of treacle
Electrolyte powder
250 g glucose powder
500 ml colostrum in plastic
   bottle (deep frozen)
1 packet of table salt.

Chapter 2

PROBLEMS OF KIDS

Before going into detailed descriptions of specific problems, it is important to familiarise the reader with some aspects of the anatomy and functioning of the unweaned kid.

The main requirements for the newborn kid are shelter, warmth and milk from its dam (colostrum). Kids are frequently born at unfavourable times of the year (springtime) when ambient temperatures are low and the risk of chilling is high and Figure 2.1 stresses the importance of these factors.

The provision of these requirements gives the kid a fighting chance to live; failure to provide any one requirement can lead to death. After birth the kid begins to use up its stores of energy and, unless that store is replenished by sucking milk, the kid becomes chilled. Cold weather accelerates the consumption of the kid's energy store, making it more urgent that the kid takes milk.

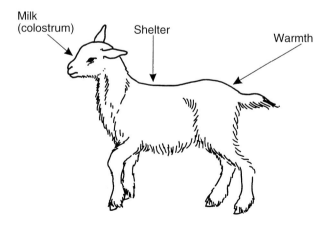

FIGURE 2.1   Basic requirements of the newborn kid

DIGESTION IN THE UNWEANED KID

The digestive process of the unweaned kid differs markedly from that of the adult goat (*see* page 74). Whereas the unweaned kid resembles a single-stomached animal such as the dog or cat, adult goats have a complex series of stomachs designed for the digestion of grass and herbage. Although the kid is born with a complete set of four stomachs, a special mechanism operates to by-pass all but the true stomach or abomasum. This mechanism is the oesophageal groove.

The Oesophageal Groove
The oesophageal groove connects the oesophagus to the abomasum as shown in Figure 2.2.

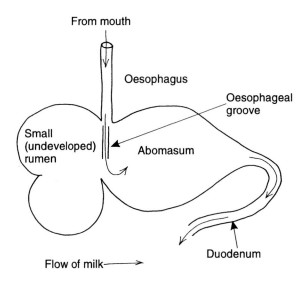

FIGURE 2.2   The position of the oesophageal groove

When the kid sucks a reflex occurs which results in the groove forming a tube (*see* Figure 2.3). Milk can then pass directly down the oesophagus to the abomasum. This mechanism avoids milk stagnating in the undeveloped rumen.

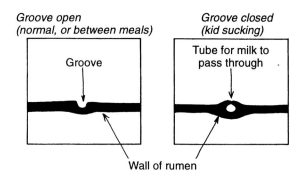

FIGURE 2.3   The kid's oesophageal groove (in section)

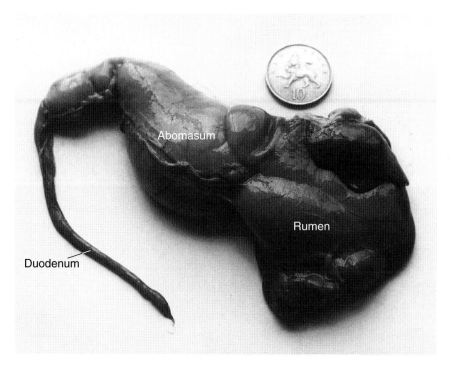

PLATE 2.1   The stomachs and duodenum of a 24-hour-old kid showing the
undeveloped rumen. Compare with the fully developed rumen,
Plate 4.3. (The coin shown measures 28mm in diameter.)

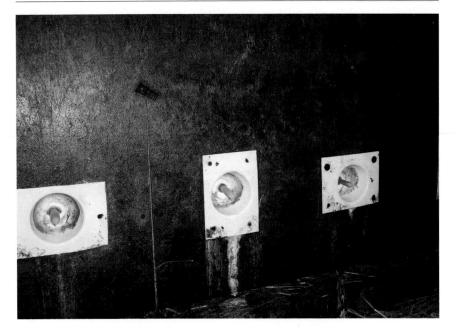

PLATE 2.2   Wall-mounted teats for kid rearing (ad-lib system)

The Oesophageal Groove Closure Reflex

It is important for goatkeepers to understand the stimuli which evoke the groove closure, and therefore avoid digestive upsets in artificially reared young kids. Whilst it is widely accepted that many substances such as milk or some salts can cause the groove to close, the 'psychological' influence may be little appreciated. Closure of the groove can occur in response to 'conditioning', even in the adult. Thus if the kid is 'conditioned' or accustomed to drinking milk soon after it sees a milk bottle, then very soon just the sight of the milk bottle causes groove closure. Similarly if the kid associates drinking milk with the rattle of certain buckets, this noise alone will stimulate groove closure after a short time. The importance of this in keeping kids healthy is obvious. Always be consistent in feeding routines. This will ensure that groove closure has occurred just before feeding, simply because the signs received by the kid are consistent each feeding time.

THE NEWBORN KID

Chilling at Birth (Hypothermia) and Starvation

As I have stressed, it is essential that the newborn kid takes in milk as soon after birth as possible. The colder the surrounding temperature, the more urgent this first drink becomes. If milk is not drunk in time, chilling or hypothermia results, because no energy is available for the kid. To check if milk has been sucked, place your hand under the abdomen of the kid and gently close you hand around the belly, the full abdomen feels like a ball whereas an empty stomach feels empty and slack.

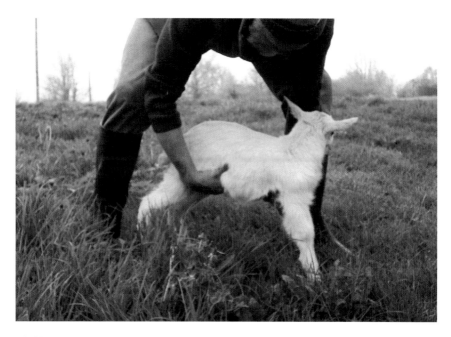

PLATE 2.3   Feeling kid's stomach for fullness

Symptoms
Shivering is the first symptom, as the kid attempts to release heat as a by-product of muscular activity. The kid walks around stiffly and aimlessly, until eventually it becomes quiet and comatose. If left it will quickly die, but if treated a large proportion of cases

will respond. Never give up with such a kid until you have tried the following course of action.

Treatment
- Dry the coat by rubbing with a warm towel.
- Put the kid into a warm place, such as by the kitchen stove or a radiator.
- Give the kid instant energy (usually a glucose solution).

Giving Glucose
Trickling fluids down the mouth of a comatose kid is dangerous, it is better first to revive the kid by warming it gently, until its body temperature is 37°C.

By stomach tube. Many shepherds and vets have a small soft rubber tube with a reservoir on the end, which is used to dose glucose solution directly into the stomach (*see* plate 2.4). These are obtainable from many farm supply dealers. The tube is introduced into the mouth over the tongue and gently pushed down the throat. It is easily done in a comatose kid but is not so easy with a fully conscious one.

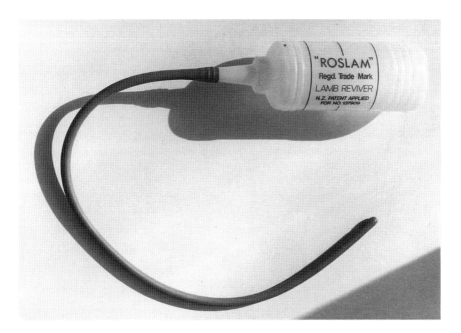

Plate 2.4   Stomach tube (lamb reviver)

By injection. In some cases your vet may use an injection in order to revive comatose kids, but many can be saved by your own efforts. Once the kid becomes conscious, it should be encouraged to take in colostrum either directly from the doe, from a bottle with a teat on it, or from a shallow container.

The temperature of the colostrum offered is vitally important, many kids will fuss and fail to drink, if it is not warm enough. A kid requires one litre of colostrum in the first 24 hours.

Many shepherds construct a 'warming box' for reviving chilled lambs, which may be useful in large goatherds. A cardboard carton is ideal (disposable) with a heat source, lamp or fan heater; take care – fire risk! The kid must obviously be checked frequently so as not to overheat.

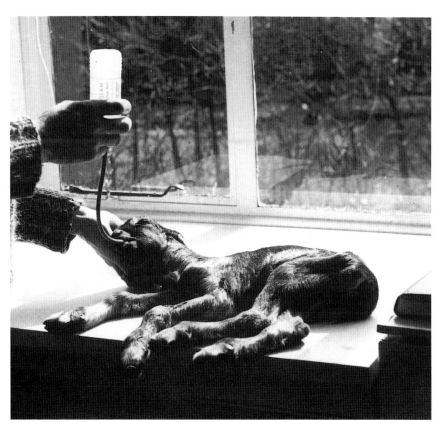

PLATE 2.5   Administration of glucose by stomach tube to a comatose kid

Developmental Abnormalities

Cleft Palate

During foetal development failure of the formation of the roof of the mouth may occur, resulting in a cleft palate (*see* plate 2.6). Problems arise when the kids attempt to suck. Because of the difficulty of forming a vacuum in the mouth, little milk is obtained during suckling. Some milk will be seen refluxing down the nose and the kid may cough and sneeze in between sucking milk.

Treatment
There is no treatment, the kids are best put down soon after birth.

Prevention
The cause is often hereditary but sometimes nutritional factors of the dam such as deficiencies or poisons may be responsible.

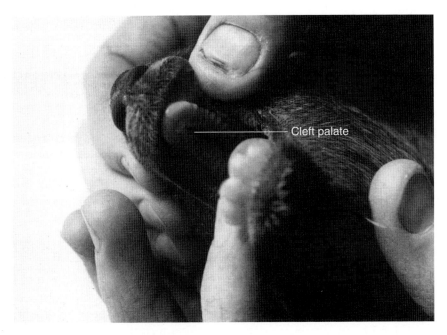

PLATE 2.6   Cleft palate in a newborn kid

YOUNG KIDS

THE MAJOR CONSIDERATIONS

- Vaccination of the dam
- Colostrum intake
- Hygiene
- Environment
- Space allowance
- Number of kids in the group
- Source of the kids
- The diet of the pregnant goat.

Vaccination of the Dam and Colostrum Intake

Measures to avoid problems with kids start prior to mating with vaccination of the doe. Protection is passed in the mother's first milk (colostrum), when the kid sucks its first meal. Colostrum has a laxative effect, helping the kid to pass its first stools (meconium), and it is rich in fat-soluble vitamins. It also contains a 'package deal' of antibodies precisely formulated for the environment of the goat. Thus, goats should be kept in the place they are due to kid for at least fourteen days prior to kidding to enable the doe to manufacture the correct range of antibodies. The next essential is to ensure that this colostrum is consumed as soon as possible, because the kid's intestine can only absorb it for a time limited to about twelve hours. Colostrum provides a very important source of energy, the kid requires about one litre in the first 24 hours. It can be stored for a year in a deep-freeze but must be defrosted slowly, not microwaved. Use a bain-marie. If goat colostrum is not available, cow colostrum can be used. The donor cow (from the same farm) can even be vaccinated with clostridial vaccine, if planned in advance, in order to provide protection to the young kids.

Hygiene

At birth the kid passes from the sterile womb to the contaminated environment of the outside world. Providing the young kid is only gradually exposed to various disease agents few problems arise. Big problems can occur, however, if hygiene is poor and colonisation of the kid's intestine by bacteria is too rapid. Thus, all utensils and fixtures with which the kid comes into contact should be as clean as possible. In general, hygiene becomes less important as the kid matures, but one must start off carefully.

Environment

Disease is rarely the simple invasion of an animal by microbes; other factors such as the environment play an important part in determining whether or not an infection causes disease. The better the conditions in which we keep our kids, the greater the microbial challenge that they can resist. The requirements for kids are a warm dry bed and good ventilation which is free from draughts. It is important to remember that kids are unable to produce as much body warmth as their parents because the kids' rumens are not functional.

Space Allowance and the Number of Kids in a Group

The space allowance of the kids is important because too little means that they are more heavily challenged by microbial agents. When large groups of kids are kept together further complications may arise, despite the fact that the space allowance is apparently adequate. Bedding must be replenished frequently, otherwise coccidiosis can occur.

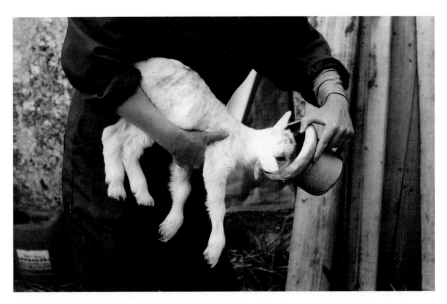

PLATE 2.7 Teaching a kid to drink: raise the hind end and use a shallow container

Many people are concerned about whether kids should be reared singly or in groups of say four or five. I feel that the benefits arising from kids of a similar age group being together, keeping each other warm and content, outweigh the disadvantages. This assumes of course that the checklist of considerations has been taken into account. We have raised many batches of fifteen or twenty kids without any problems.

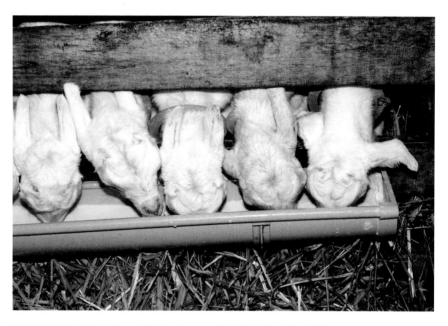

PLATE 2.8   Plastic guttering is excellent for feeding kids

Source of Kids
If kids are purchased from outside sources, i.e. other breeders, problems may arise. As stated earlier, the colostral antibody is for a specific environment. It does not necessarily give the correct protection for a new environment. Also, each kid has its own range of micro-organisms and these may be very different from those of its new pen-mates; this may cause disease outbreaks. Stress arising from transportation and mixing is also relevant in bought-in kids. In many circumstances it may be better to isolate new kids from the resident goats until they are old enough to mix out at grass.

The Diet of the Pregnant Goat
This must be adequate in quantity and quality in order to nourish a healthy kid.

DIARRHOEA

The most common disease problems of kids are those where the main symptom is that of diarrhoea (scour). Most of the checklist given previously will have a bearing upon the occurrence of diarrhoea. The types of disease agents involved are many and varied, including *E. coli* bacteria and rotavirus (*see* the list below).

When investigating the problem in kids your vet may well take samples for laboratory investigation or even send off dead kids to the lab. Whilst this is being done the goatkeeper's efforts should be directed to general hygiene and avoiding the predisposing causes outlined in the previous pages.

Some Agents Associated with Diarrhoea in Kids

Escherichia coli	*Eimeria* spp.
Salmonella spp.	*Rotavirus*
Clostridium welchii	*Herpes virus*
Cryptosporidium parvum	*Coronavirus*

DIETARY SCOUR

Diarrhoea frequently develops simply because changes in feeding have been made or too much food has been offered to the kid. The change in food has the effect of modifying the conditions within the intestines perhaps, for example, by altering the acidity or alkalinity. Micro-organisms such as bacteria grow at different rates in different situations and the changes will favour one type, allowing them to flourish at the expense of others. This results in large amounts of toxin being produced which irritates the gut wall causing it to lose water and salts. This is seen as diarrhoea.

Many of these bacteria such as *E. coli* are present in healthy kids and they only get out of hand when conditions change (*see* below). Preventing this type of scour depends upon avoiding drastic feed changes. Two situations in which I have seen this problem are: firstly, a rapid change to milk replacer and secondly, incorrectly made-up milk replacer. When using milk replacer always add the quantity of water given in the directions on the bag.

The danger of these upsets is that they predispose to enterotoxaemia (*see* page 89). (*See also* DIETARY SCOUR IN ADULT GOATS, page 88.)

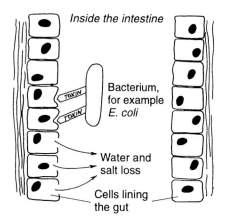

Inside the intestine

Bacterium, for example *E. coli*

Water and salt loss

Cells lining the gut

FIGURE 2.4   Bacterial toxins acting on the intestines to cause loss of fluid

E.Coli

Some *E.coli* can cause severe diarrhoea in young animals and human infants.

The isolation of *Escherichia coli* from faecal samples can be confusing to the goatkeeper because there are two classes of *E. coli*.

1. Normal flora – normally non-pathogenic
2. Pathogenic.

The pathogens tend to be identified by serogroups and have numbers such as 0145 ascribed to them. These bacteria can be further subdivided according to how they exert their harmful effects such as, enteropathogenic or enterotoxigenic. Your vet will help with interpretation of such laboratory reports.

Treatment.
This will be mainly aimed at rehydration using oral electrolytes and possibly by intravenous injections. Occasionally antibiotics will be given depending upon laboratory findings.

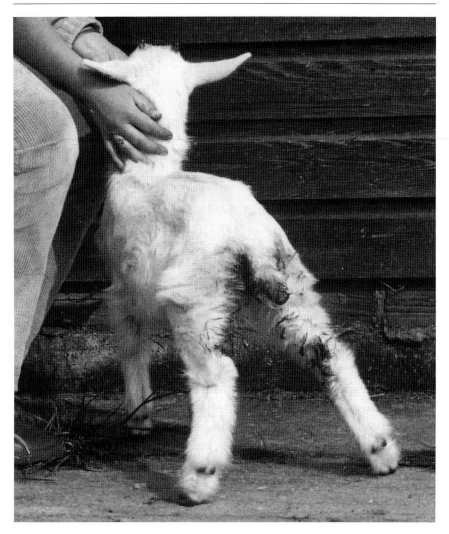

PLATE 2.9   Kid with dietary scour

SALMONELLOSIS

Infection by many of the 1600 serotypes or strains of *Salmonella* organisms can occur in goats. Many cases have been reported overseas, but it is seen only rarely in the United Kingdom and North America. Serotypes have included *S. typhimurium*, one which can cause food poisoning in human beings. Infection with

Salmonella organisms does not necessarily result in disease, there are many healthy goats shedding this germ in their droppings. Trigger factors such as stress can precipitate the disease of salmonellosis.

Symptoms
Kids are generally the most severely affected, with symptoms including diarrhoea, high temperature, blood poisoning and, often, death. Because of the acute nature of the disease the diarrhoea is often blood-tinged or even black.

Prevention
Avoiding all the situations which impose stress on the kids is the surest way to stay clear of the disease; among these situations are irregular feeding, draughts and long journeys. The problem cannot be controlled by vaccination because there are so many different strains. In adult goats salmonellosis is rare but may occur when goats are exposed to the stressors mentioned above. In such cases the symptoms start with diarrhoea, weakness and the goats progressively remain lying down. Deaths may well occur.

Treatment
The severe nature of this disease in kids will dictate that the goatkeeper seeks the assistance of his vet. Treatment must be started early and your vet will probably use fluid replacement therapy and possibly antibiotics. The proportion of deaths among kids affected by this condition can be very high. Nursing is particularly important in determining survival.

COCCIDIOSIS

Diarrhoea is one of the main symptoms of coccidiosis. However, as the problem is most intimately connected with housing conditions I have included it in Chapter 3 (*see* COCCIDIOSIS, page 67).

ENTEROTOXAEMIA AND DYSENTERY
(caused by Clostridium perfringens types B C and D)

Vaccination of the doe is especially important in avoiding the problem of enterotoxaemia in kids. Enterotoxaemia caused by

Clostridium perfringens type D, is a killer disease in herds not using routine clostridial vaccination. The clostridia are a family of bacteria, the most well known member of which causes tetanus (lockjaw) in humans and animals.

Enterotoxaemia can affect goats of all ages, but tends to be more lethal in young kids. The bacteria are commonly found in the soil and most animals will have them in their intestines. It is, therefore, unrealistic to think of keeping goats free from them. The lethal action of these organisms is that they release toxins into the blood which give rise to shock and nervous symptoms. There are specific receptor sites such as the heart, brain and intestine upon which the toxins are targeted.

Dysentery in kids results from an infection with Clostridium perfringens type C. It generally affects very young kids, causing diarrhoea with blood in it or even sudden death. The toxins released from the multiplying organisms in the intestine, cause inflammation and death of the lining of the gut.

Prevention
It is possible to increase the immunity of the kid to the clostridia. This is successfully achieved by vaccinating the doe before pregnancy and letting her pass the protection on to the kid by way of the colostrum. Avoiding the conditions which allow the organism to proliferate in the intestines and release their toxins is equally important. Sudden changes in the type of food or quantity fed will aid this proliferation. Changes in the kids' feed must therefore be gradual, and up to a week should be taken to change from one type to another. It is also important to avoid engorgement by kids, for example after they have become excessively hungry.

All goats should be vaccinated against this disease at least once a year, preferably twice. When vaccinating, great care should be taken to avoid injecting into the muscle. The correct site is under the skin. For the primary vaccination, give two doses with an interval of 4 weeks. Vaccinate before breeding and avoid vaccinating during pregnancy. Check the manufacturer's directions.

Symptoms
The symptoms of enterotoxaemia are sudden in their onset and include depression and a drunken appearance. As the disease progresses the animal becomes unable to stand and lies on its side making paddling movements. Very watery diarrhoea may be

seen, depending upon the severity of the condition. I have seen kids die within an hour of displaying these symptoms. With type C, bloody diarrhoea (dysentery) is the main symptom.

Treatment
Treatment of this condition is rarely satisfactory, but your veterinary surgeon may try giving the sick kid specific antisera. It is often more valuable to use the antisera on other members of the group for the purpose of prevention. Some vets report successful treatment using sulphonamides by mouth, in adult goats. General treatment is directed against shock. Recent research work underlines the susceptibility of the kid to type D. Post mortem findings were haemorrhagic entero-colitis (inflammation of the small and large intestines). Death occurred rapidly and treatment was futile.

TREATMENT OF DIARRHOEA

The production of loose faeces is generally an indication that the intestinal system has been damaged and, like most damaged organs, requires resting until repair has been carried out. The function of repair is carried out by the body's own system, but ensuring that the intestine is rested requires the goatkeeper to restrict the kids' intake of food.

Generally, restricting the food for one day will alleviate many scour problems. Only small quantities of food must be offered for the subsequent three days, otherwise the good work will be wasted. For unweaned kids, restriction to only half the normal milk intake is recommended, following twenty-four hours of no milk. In this first twenty-four hours electrolytes (salts) should be offered to the kid at about 39°C (a litre minimum, divided over three feeds). If the milk is restricted then make it up to the normal daily volume with electrolyte solution. Feed the milk and electrolyte separately. Do not dilute the milk. The electrolytes can arrive as sachets (requiring water to be added) or liquid; always make sure you obtain some from your vet and hold them in your medicine cupboard. They are inexpensive and yet very effective. Some names of commercial products available are Effydral and Lectade.

Severe cases of diarrhoea, when the faeces resemble dirty water or when blood is observed in the droppings, probably require help from your vet, who will probably prescribe electrolytes by injection (intravenous drip). Some cases of scour in young kids require antibiotic treatment if septicaemia (blood poisoning) is suspected.

CRYPTOSPORIDIOSIS

This protozoan parasite disease is reported world-wide causing diarrhoea in young kids, calves and lambs. The disease is caused by *Cryptosporidium parvum*. It is a zoonose, meaning it affects humans as well.

It causes a watery diarrhoea in young kids under a month old and may spread to affect all the kids in the group. The parasite invades the cells lining the small intestine causing damage and subsequent diarrhoea. Infection spreads quickly from kid to kid. Infected buildings are not easily disinfected and formalin solution or ammonia based disinfectants are required. Hot water (60°C) together with detergent is also effective. After cleaning and disinfecting the building try and open it up to sunlight.

Treatment and prevention.
There are no useful drugs to treat this disease but Decoquinate (Forum Products Ltd) is claimed to prevent it if used before a challenge. The aim of treatment is to rehydrate the scouring kids, thus electrolytes are required. (*See* TREATMENT OF DIARRHOEA page 38.) Try to avoid buying-in kids but if you do have to, keep them separate from your other stock. Try to use an all-in all-out policy for kid rearing. Apply similar husbandry practices as for coccidiosis with an emphasis on providing a clean environment into which the new-born kids can be placed.

SEPTICAEMIA

Septicaemia or blood poisoning can follow a simple case of diarrhoea. If the antibodies that protect the intestine from invasion are overcome, bacteria can cross through into the bloodstream. Kids that have had colostrum would normally be able to defend themselves against such an invasion because in these cases the antibody from the colostrum is present in the bloodstream and acts by 'mopping-up' the invading bacteria. Should the kid have missed its colostrum the blood poisoning rapidly takes a hold and the kid becomes very ill within twelve hours. The symptoms are those of a sick kid with a high temperature and severe

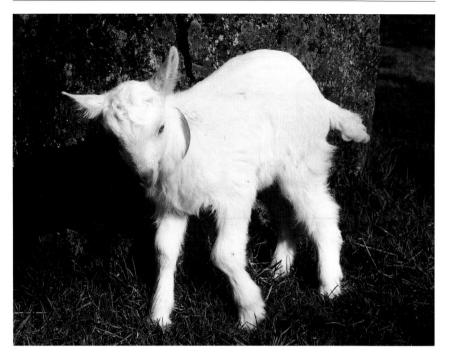

PLATE 2.10   Kid with joint ill

diarrhoea. Sometimes the septicaemia develops so rapidly that diarrhoea is not noticed.

Treatment and prevention
Antibiotics and fluid therapy can save many of the kids but prevention rests upon the simple rule of ensuring that all kids take in colostrum.

COLIC

Colic can affect young kids especially when dietary changes are made. Introducing milk replacer or mixing it up at the wrong concentration can precipitate colic. Spasm and excess gas production is caused in the bowel, giving rise to pain.

Symptoms
The kid is restless, cries out and tends to stand either with its

back arched or with its hind feet placed well back. Its nose and mouth may feel cold.

Treatment
In mild cases the pain quickly passes and the kid returns to normal within hours. Severe cases may require drugs to relieve the pain. Buscopan (Boehringer) is a relaxant, given by injection. Liquid paraffin (5–15 ml) given by mouth may help.

NAVEL ILL AND JOINT ILL

These diseases are generally caused by dirty environments. Throughout pregnancy the umbilical cord connects the kid to the placenta, enabling it to receive nutrients from the doe. Once detached at birth, the cord rapidly dries out and shrivels, leaving a scar of attachment, the navel. Immediately after birth, the fleshy navel is open to infection and it contains blood vessels

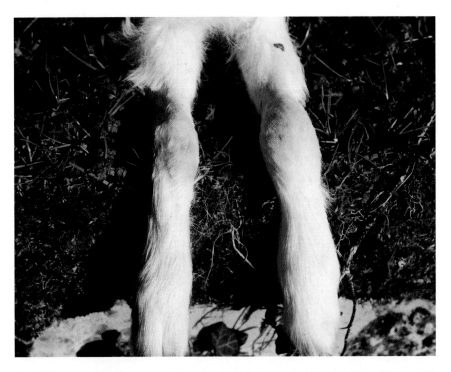

PLATE 2.11   Swollen carpal joint on the left-hand side of a kid with joint ill
              (right-hand side of plate)

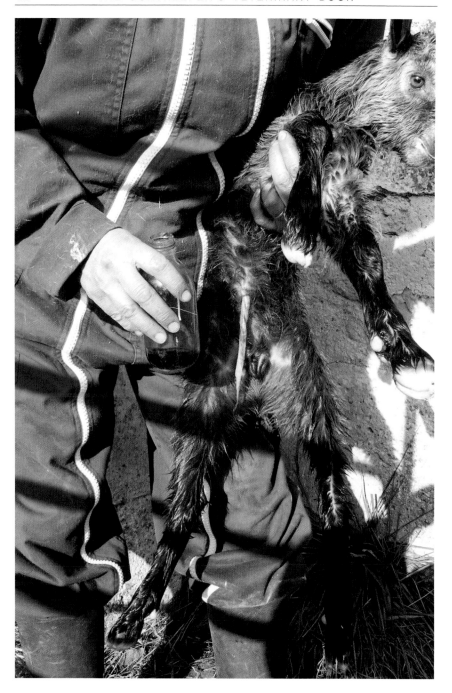

PLATE 2.12   Navel prior to dipping

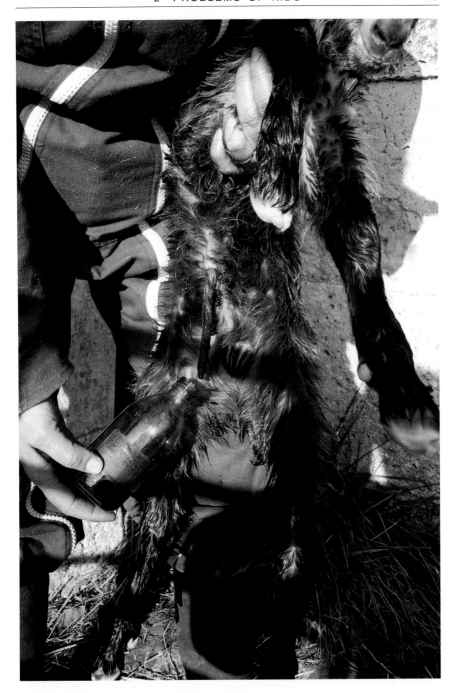

PLATE 2.13   Navel after dipping in tincture of iodine

which, if infected, can result in an infected liver or possibly blood poisoning. Infection may also spread to the joints via the blood, causing 'joint ill'.

Symptoms
The young kid with this condition has a swollen, painful navel which may look red and 'angry'. The kid is commonly off its food and may or may not have swollen joints, if the condition has progressed to joint ill. More usually the joint involvement becomes evident after some weeks.

Treatment
Navel ill is generally treatable, and your vet will probably prescribe antibiotic injections. The area around the navel should be cleaned with antiseptic iodine, crusty scabs removed by soaking and any pockets of pus drained. Joint ill tends to leave badly damaged joints and it may well be better not to embark on a course of treatment; euthanasia may be preferable.

Prevention
The goatkeeper should aim to prevent this problem by providing hygienic conditions at kidding, and in the opinion of the author, a clean grass paddock is equally desirable to a kidding box. The kidding box should be well strawed up and the navel could be dressed soon after birth. For dressing navels (i.e. putting antiseptic substances on to the raw cord), sprays, iodine solutions or powders can be supplied by your vet. Tincture of iodine is ideal.

TETANUS

Infection of open wounds by the bacterium Clostridium tetani results in tetanus (lockjaw). It is not common in goats, but it may affect young kids. As with enterotoxaemia, the organisms are present in the soil in a special form known as a 'spore'. In this form the bacterium can survive for many years, always being present, ready to infect deep wounds. The germs multiply in the wound releasing toxins which are harmful to the nerves. The toxins travel up the nerve trunk to the spinal cord and brain, where they cause constant excitability of the nerves. This results in the muscles contracting all the time, and therefore the goat walks stiffly.

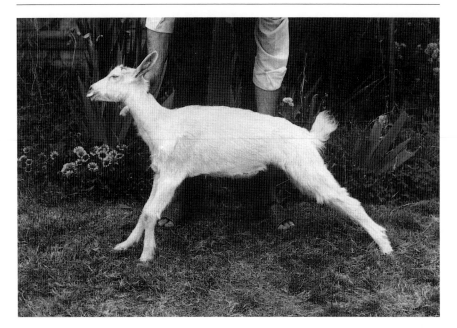

PLATE 2.14   Tetanus in a kid

Symptoms
A general increase in muscle stiffness is seen, causing an
unsteady gait. The third eyelid begins to extend over the eye and
the animal looks 'anxious'. The symptoms get progressively
worse and convulsions may occur. The goat dies because it is
unable to breathe.

Treatment
Goats can be treated with penicillin and antisera, but response is
poor.

Prevention
Avoid dirty conditions when wounds such as castration cuts are
present and likely to become infected.

Vaccination of all goats is cheap and effective; the vaccine is
normally included in the multiple vaccines for enterotoxaemia.
In the UK, Lambivac (Intervet UK Ltd) and Tetanus Toxoid
Concentrated (Intervet UK Ltd) are both licensed for use in
goats.

Young kids receive protection from their mother's colostrum, providing that she is vaccinated each year. This maternal protection will persist until the kid is twelve weeks of age. Kids retained for rearing should therefore be vaccinated at about three months. Tetanus Toxoid (vaccine) can be given on its own.

ENZOOTIC ATAXIA (SWAYBACK)

This condition, causing lack of hind limb co-ordination, has been relatively rarely recorded in kids; it is similar to 'swayback' in lambs.

Symptoms
The symptoms are of weak kids, unable to rise or 'swaying' at the back end. They are associated with poor development of the nerve fibres, resulting from a deficiency of copper in the diet of the dam during pregnancy. Because the individual attention given to goats during pregnancy is generally superior to that given to sheep, this condition is less likely to occur in kids. Nevertheless it does still occur in the UK. Owners suspecting swayback should contact their veterinary surgeon to confirm their suspicions. Reports suggest that the condition is incurable. Advice about future prevention should be sought, in order to avoid the problem in next year's kids.

CONTRACTED TENDONS

Quite commonly kids are born with contracted tendons of the forelegs.

This results in the kid walking on its fetlock joints. Frequently the condition resolves itself as the kid starts to put weight on the hoof and hence stretches the tendons. Sometimes bandages and splints are required in order to compel the kid to put weight on the hoof.

Two inherited conditions can also give rise to kids being born with contracted tendons. A congenital defect in Australian Angora goats, with complex inheritance patterns, generally results in both sides being affected. The other condition affects Anglo-nubian kids in many parts of the world including Australia and North America. It is caused by a genetic condition called beta-mannosidosis. Diagnosis can be confirmed by blood testing.

Control

In inherited conditions, changes in the breeding lines would be necessary to prevent such kids being produced.

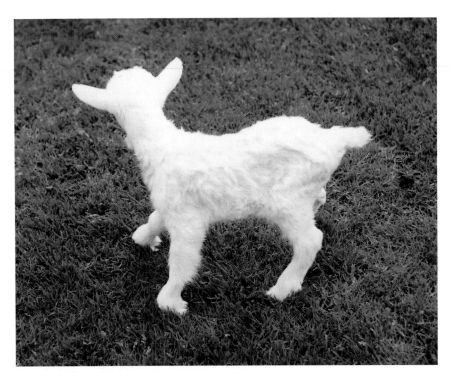

PLATE 2.15   Kid with contracted tendons

DIPHTHERIA (ULCERATIVE STOMATITIS)

This problem occurs very rarely in young goats. It is essentially a disease of dirty conditions and is generally seen in housed kids.

The organism most commonly isolated from infected kids is Fusiformis necrophorus. This germ is universally present around animals, and infection enters through cuts. It is thought that rough food and teething can be responsible for cuts in the mouth, and in one outbreak all the affected goats had diphtheria in either the mouth, tongue or throat.

Symptoms
These will depend upon the area involved but salivation, noisy breathing and smelly breath are common observations.

Treatment
Good response to treatment can be expected from using anti-bacterial drugs such as sulphonamides. Your veterinary surgeon will prescribe something suitable.

Prevention
Hygiene in the rearing of kids is the key to preventing the disease. Cleanliness of feed and water containers is especially important.

CAPRINE ARTHRITIS ENCEPHALITIS VIRUS (CAE)
(*See* page 226)

ROUTINE PROCEDURES

THE DISBUDDING OF KIDS

Horned goats are a danger and a nuisance. Many owners of horned kids have the horns removed when they are about three to five days old. The technique is termed 'disbudding' and it is a fairly simple job when the goat is young. Conversely, removal of the horns of adult goats is a major operation and should only be carried out in the winter when flies are not active.

Horn buds can be removed either by using caustic chemicals or by burning. Burning is by far the most satisfactory method, and the procedure must be carried out by a veterinary surgeon.

Procedure
The kid should preferably be prevented from sucking for four hours before disbudding. A general anaesthetic is preferable to local anaesthesia. The hair surrounding the horn bud is clipped away, and some suggest the use of cosmetic hair removers to accomplish this step. Using a very hot iron, your veterinary surgeon will burn away the horn bud taking care to burn all the skin around the base. Recovery from a general anaesthetic can

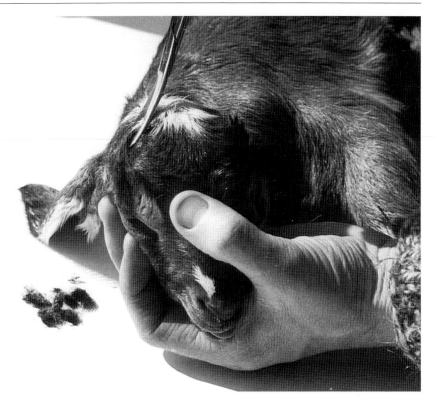

PLATE 2.16   Clipping hair prior to disbudding

take some hours, depending upon the drugs used. Ensure that the mouth is lower than the rest of the body, to allow saliva to drain from the mouth.

Notes for Veterinarians

Fatalities have occurred following disbudding. Brain damage can occur if the disbudding iron is left in contact with the skull for prolonged periods, so use a very hot iron for a short period.

Probably the most widely used methods of anaesthesia for disbudding kids are:

- *Halothane/oxygen* by mask. With 2–3% halothane the kid is anaesthetised in about 3 minutes. N.B. Remember to remove the oxygen supply whilst burning.

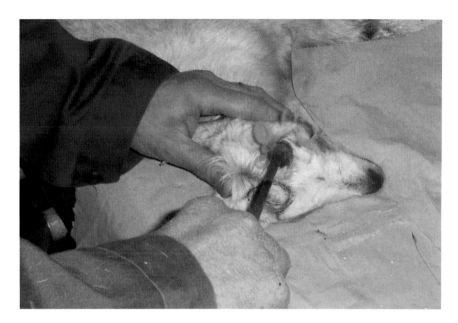

PLATE 2.17   Disbudding the anaesthetised kid

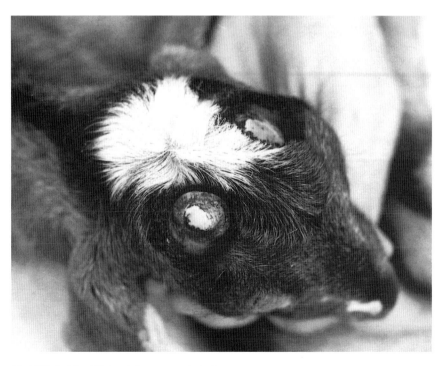

PLATE 2.18   Disbudding completed

- *Rompun* (Bayer), a sedative/pain killer used in conjunction with local anaesthesia. 0.10 mls of Rompun for an average 4–5 day old kid. (Prolonged recovery – avoid in cold weather.)
- *Saffan* (Schering-Plough) can be given by intramuscular injection, usually in the quadriceps muscle mass, at a dose rate of 0.75 ml/kg. The dose can be divided and given in each leg to reduce pain. The kid is anaesthetised in 5 minutes and recovery takes 30–40 minutes. The intravenous route may also be used.

CASTRATION OF MALE KIDS

Sometimes it may be necessary to neuter male kids. Owners may wish to rear an animal for pulling a goat-cart or even just to make a non-smelling pet. When rearing male kids for meat production it is probably best not to castrate them because a better carcase results from an entire male. This may not be possible if the males have to be reared with females because they become sexually active from four months of age. It is also advisable to have them castrated if the rearing period extends through to September – the breeding season. If this happens, the entire males go off their food and do not put on weight, delaying the time for slaughter.

Methods
The testicles must be 'inactivated', either by removing them or by destroying them where they lie. Methods 1 and 2 below are normally carried out under general or local anaesthesia. Readers are advised to seek advice as to the laws of their country concerning castration. In the UK it may be carried out, without an anaesthetic, under the age of 2 months.

1. Removal using a scalpel (surgical castration)
The scrotum is incised, the testicles exposed and pulled out. The spermatic cord and the wound are dressed with antibiotic powder or cream.

2. The Burdizzo
Using a special instrument (*see* plate 2.20) the spermatic cord and blood vessels are squeezed between two metal jaws. The effect is to prevent blood reaching the testicles so that they gradually wither away, becoming small and inactive. After several weeks the testicles should be re-examined in order to determine

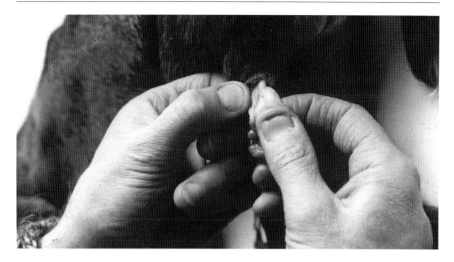

PLATE 2.19   Surgical castration

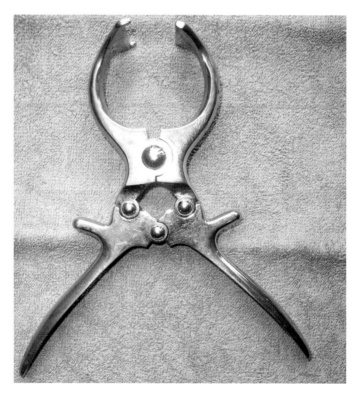

PLATE 2.20   Burdizzo

whether or not the operation was successful. If the method worked the testicles should be small and hard. At this stage all testicular hormone and semen production ceases.

3. The Rubber Ring Method

A similar technique to (2) is to place a special elastic band around the neck of the scrotum, thus restricting the blood supply to both the testicles and the scrotum. The withered scrotum and testicles eventually drop off about two weeks later. Though effective, this method gives rise to considerable discomfort to the kid and, in the view of many veterinary surgeons, is inhumane. This procedure must be carried out under one week of age (in the UK).

EUTHANASIA OF KIDS

Surplus male kids can be a problem to goatkeepers with limited accommodation. Fortunately, there is an increasing demand for kid meat and there are now outlets for people wishing to dispose of these young kids. If there is no outlet for the kids, a licensed slaughterman should be consulted. Alternatively, your veterinary surgeon will 'put them to sleep' for you, using injections.

Chapter 3

DISEASES ASSOCIATED WITH HOUSED GOATS

RESPIRATORY DISEASES

WHAT IS A RESPIRATORY DISEASE?

A respiratory disease is any condition affecting the breathing apparatus of the goat. This includes the nose, trachea (windpipe), bronchi, and lungs. It may also involve the pleura or membranes which surround the lungs. The respiratory system of the goat is illustrated in Figure 3.1.

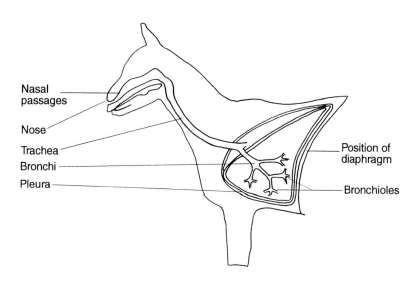

FIGURE 3.1 Breathing apparatus of the goat

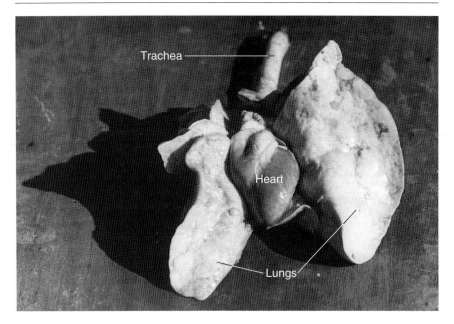

PLATE 3.1   Lungs and heart of the goat

BREATHING IN THE HEALTHY GOAT

There is one substance that is present in abundance on this planet, and that is fresh air. It is because of this abundant supply of air that the majority of us keep healthy for most of the time. Animals breathe in order to take oxygen into their lungs and to allow waste gas (carbon dioxide) out. The oxygen is vital for all the tissues of the body. The lungs are the organs that bring about the exchange of oxygen from the air into our blood, and the exhalation of carbon dioxide.

Figure 3.2 illustrates the basic function of the lungs: gaseous exchange. When the goat inhales and exhales, water droplets and micro-organisms are also passing into and out of the goat's respiratory system. The water arises from the moist lung surface and the micro-organisms from all parts of the breathing apparatus such as the trachea, bronchioles and larynx. The breathing apparatus of a healthy goat is colonised by many different types of bacteria, viruses and other micro-organisms. This is normal and natural. In most circumstances the goat remains healthy because it produces antibodies, and because it possesses a complex system which keeps the bacteria and viruses under control.

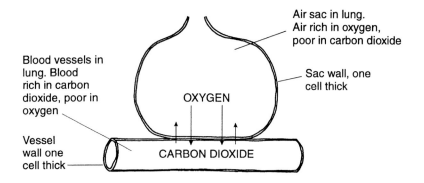

FIGURE 3.2   Gaseous exchange in the lung

THE FACTORS PREDISPOSING TO RESPIRATORY DISEASE

These factors are:

- A shared air space with other goats, especially goats from another farm
- Poor ventilation
- Age of the housed goats
- Stress, such as housing or temperature change.

A Shared Air Space
When a goat in a field breathes out, the bacteria and viruses which are exhaled in that breath are soon dispersed. The situation inside a small house, however, is very different. The micro-organisms and water vapour are not easily diluted, so they have a profound effect on the air inside, making it humid and laden with many micro-organisms. These micro-organisms are then inhaled by other goats. It must also be remembered that the water vapour will have altered the relative humidity of the air. This is thought to adversely affect the tissues of the respiratory tract, reducing their defensive capabilities. The combination of these changes – heavy doses of micro-organisms, and the effect on the lungs and trachea – may precipitate respiratory disease.

Ventilation
The principle of ventilation is to ensure that the air within the goat house is changed regularly. This provides fresh air for the goats to breathe and removes the foul air containing the micro-

organisms. It is always better to provide more rather than less ventilation. Owners' fears about chilling their goats are unfounded, providing that direct draughts are excluded. Air should circulate freely in the goat house, but you should ensure 'cosy' areas where the goats can be protected from draughts by solid partitions. Remember that the rumen is like a central heating system keeping adult goats warm; kids do not possess this heat source until they are of weaning age.

Age of the Goats

Another important consideration is the age of the animal in the goat house. Older animals tend to have experienced many bacteria and viruses in the normal course of their lives. Young kids and goatlings are less fortunate. Often the first time they experience a new type of virus is in a goat house where the dose can be high, and they succumb to infection. Thus one must be particularly careful about providing the correct environmental conditions for young goats if respiratory disease is to be avoided.

Stress

As already discussed, many changes stress goats, for example, housing and mixing or transport.

SIGNS AND SYMPTOMS OF RESPIRATORY DISEASE

The most common type of respiratory disease seen in housed goats is an infection of some part or even the whole of the system. Other less common diseases include allergies, deficiencies, cancers and so on. The reasons for the high frequency of infections are the predisposing conditions already described. Of the many types of agents that can be involved, most are viruses and bacteria. For example, one study revealed fifteen different types of bacteria in goat pneumonias. Viruses have the property of being able to invade healthy cells and they tend to commence the disease processes. They damage the tissues, leaving them vulnerable to attack by bacteria and mycoplasma. The symptoms we see are simply a reflection of the area damaged. For example, an infection of the nose results in a discharge being produced from the nostrils, and symptoms of rapid breathing may be a sign of pneumonia. Similarly, an infection of the windpipe or of the bronchi tends to stimulate coughing. This cough reflex is unfortunately the commonest method by which this type of disease passes from one goat to the next. A coughing or sneezing goat produces tiny water droplets containing micro-organisms. These airborne particles are then just the right size to enter the trachea and lungs of any other goats kept in the same building. Once coughing starts, it usually spreads quickly to affect other animals. The disease spread will have occurred even before the goatkeeper has heard the first cough.

MILD UPPER RESPIRATORY TRACT INFECTIONS

These are commonly seen when large groups of young goats are kept together in badly ventilated buildings. The symptoms include coughing, nasal discharge, and raised body temperatures.

This is less commonly seen in closed herds, more common with bought-in animals.

Action to be taken
Provide plenty of fresh air and watch carefully for goats going off their food. Any goat that refuses food requires veterinary attention. These goats should be penned off from the main group and given special nursing attention.

It may be necessary to provide areas free from draughts, by using straw bales for goats to shelter behind. These can be renewed frequently. Never be concerned about letting in too much air. Other measures which may be helpful are avoiding dry, dusty food, and reducing the dust from excessively dry bedding materials.

Prevention
Ensure that all kids receive adequate colostrum immediately after birth, so that they are provided with protective antibodies.

- Always ensure adequate ventilation. As a rule of thumb, goat houses should be dry and not dripping with condensation. Goats can withstand cold environments, so long as they are not draughty.
- Try to keep the bedding dry so that it does not increase the relative humidity of the house.
- If possible, avoid mixing young goats (two to eight months) which come from different rearing places. Avoid a common air space for adults and young animals.
- The pasteurella bacteria are commonly associated with

respiratory disease in ruminants. Vaccines to control pneumonic pasteurellosis are available for sheep but they are not licensed for goats. In some circumstances your vet may recommend them. They are used on goats in countries such as France 'off label', for example, Pastobov (Merial).

Pneumonia

A better name to describe an infection of the lung would be pneumonitis, but it is traditionally referred to as pneumonia. This can result from a serious upper respiratory tract infection or possibly from drenching a goat incorrectly. In any event this condition is serious and should receive skilled attention quickly. The symptoms are those of a sick goat which refuses food, probably has an elevated temperature, coughs and breathes rapidly. Your veterinary surgeon will probably prescribe antibacterial drugs and other aids to remove the fluids from the lungs. Simple first-aid treatment includes the recommendations given under 'mild respiratory infections'. Water and food should be offered at a suitable height, not on the floor where the animal has to bend down to eat or drink. Both *Pasteurella haemolytica* and *P. multocida* have been isolated from such cases.

Drenching Pneumonia
This follows the accidental pouring of fluids into the windpipe and lungs of a goat undergoing medication. It may also result from force-feeding a kid from a bucket. Symptoms usually develop a day or so following the drenching and the course of the disease can be fatal. Your veterinary surgeon will advise you on the best course of action to take.

Mycoplasma
The mycoplasma could be considered to be small bacterium without a cell wall. They do not persist for long outside of the animal host (up to 14 days at ambient temperature). They cause significant goat respiratory disease in Continental Europe; outbreaks of coughing occur in young and old. Four strains of mycoplasma are involved in mycoplasmal disease in Europe. *Mycoplasma mycoides mycoides (LC)*, *Mycoplasma capricolum capricolum*, *Mycoplasma putrefaciens* and *Mycoplasma agalactia*.

These are not a recorded problem in the UK. The problems are generally introduced into clean herds by carrier animals.

OTHER CONDITIONS

Many other conditions manifest themselves through symptoms such as coughing or rapid breathing; an example would be an allergy. The frequency of their occurrence, however, is so low that it would be pointless to detail them in a book such as this. Your veterinary surgeon will help you in this situation.

Lungworm
It may happen that housed goats develop lungworm, resulting from an infestation gained while at pasture. (*See* LUNGWORM, page 117.)

THE FLOOR AND FOOT CONDITIONS

LAMENESS AND HOOF CARE

An important problem found in goats kept in houses is that of lameness. Frequently the cause of the lameness is associated with the nature of the floor or bed. When given a choice, goats tend to prefer dry surfaces to walk upon; indeed the habitat of the mountain goat is firm craggy rocks. Dry abrasive surfaces are ideal for the goat's hoof, which continuously produces horn in the anticipation that it will be worn away.

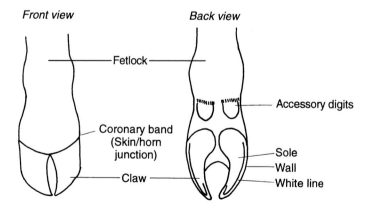

FIGURE 3.3   Anatomy of a goat's foot

Normal Horn Growth

Wall horn is produced from the skin/horn junction of the coronary band, and the horn works its way down until it comes into wear with the ground. Horn is also produced to cover the sole, but this should not be in contact with the ground. In short the weight of the goat should be borne on the edge of the wall horn which surrounds the hoof. (*See* Figure 3.4.)

FIGURE 3.4   *The weight-bearing area of a goat's hoof*

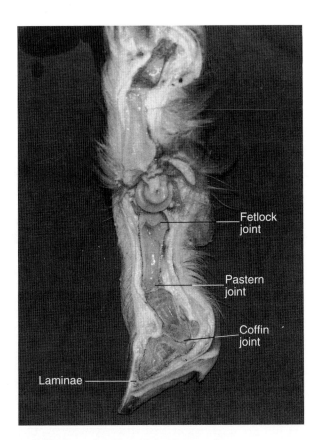

PLATE 3.2   Section through one claw

Principles of Hoof Care

Because most goats do not spend enough time walking on dry, abrasive surfaces the owner must pare away the excess horn. If this is not done, incorrect stress is placed upon the hoof, causing cracking of the horn. Stones may also become embedded in the fold of horn. Plate 3.3 shows the hoof before and after paring.

The aim of paring is to remove the surplus wall horn that tends to bend under the sole and impede normal action. Paring can be carried out using hoof shears or a hoof knife.

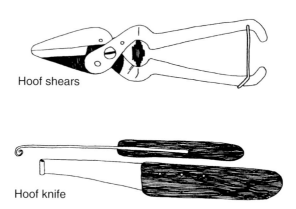

Hoof shears

Hoof knife

FIGURE 3.5   Hoof care equipment

Goats Kept on Deep Bedding

Work with cattle has revealed a great deal of information about the causes of lameness in hoofed animals, which is directly applicable to goats. One important aspect is the dryness or wetness of the floor. Ideally, as I have suggested, housed goats should be kept on a hard surface with access to a bed of straw or similar soft material. Many systems, however, do not allow this and goats can be successfully raised on deep straw bedding. In this situation there is no wear on the hoof horn and attention must be paid to paring as described in the preceding section.

Another important aspect is the effect of moisture on the hoof. Very wet bedding contains enzymes which break down the cement between the layers of horn. This predisposes to the entry of bacteria and subsequent infections developing in the hoof. These infections are termed white line abscesses. Lack of exercise is also detrimental to the hooves of goats kept standing in

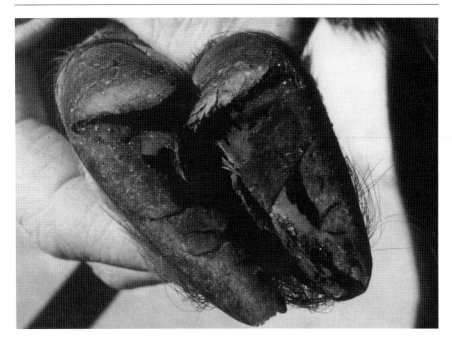

PLATE 3.3   Hoof before paring (above) and after (below)

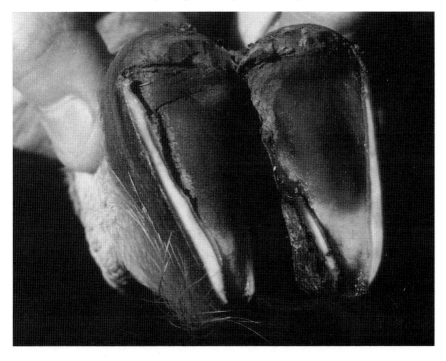

very wet conditions for long periods. In this situation the blood supply to the horn is reduced, resulting in poor growth.

Remember that lameness from any cause reduces milk yield, and hence profitability. After discussion with your vet, owners who experience a high incidence of lameness could contemplate bathing the hooves of their goats in either 10 per cent zinc sulphate solution or 3 per cent formalin solution. These solutions have the dual effect of destroying bacteria around the hoof and hardening the horn. Smaller quantities of either substance can be made up and applied to each hoof individually. Avoid splashing these solutions on to the skin or eyes, and do not leave the goats standing in formalin solution for longer than two or three minutes. Goat owners will realise that forcing goats to get their feet wet is not easy. This is a very practical problem with using foot baths.

Summary of Measures to Avoid Lameness in Housed Goats

- Pay constant attention to feet paring. (Make sure all parings are removed or burnt.)
- Provide as dry a bed as possible, with good drainage.
- If possible provide an area of dry concrete, where the goats can spend part of the day.
- Bathe feet in either 3% formalin (walk through) or stand in 10% zinc sulphate solution if required.
- Exercise daily.
- Vaccinate (only if necessary) (see FOOTROT, page 124).

SOME SPECIFIC CAUSES OF LAMENESS

CAE (CAPRINE ARTHRITIS ENCEPHALITIS VIRUS) OR BIG KNEE
(See page 226.)

FOOTROT

Although classically a problem of grazing animals in the summer time, footrot does occur when goats are bedded on straw in winter. If the conditions are warm and wet, the bacterium *Fusiformis necrophorus* can survive to be spread from one goat to the next. (See FOOTROT, page 124.)

LAMINITIS

The laminae are the sensitive tissues which lie below the layer of horn which covers the hoof (*see* plate 3.2). When these tissues are inflamed they become extremely painful, a condition described as laminitis.

Symptoms
Laminitis, like many diseases, can be either very severe or very mild, with all grades in between. Characteristically the goat appears uncomfortable, or severely lame on all its feet, especially the fore feet. The feet can feel hot when touched owing to the inflammation below the horn, and the goat's temperature is elevated. This condition arises in goats receiving heavy concentrate rations and in cases of over-eating (for example, when the goat gains access to the concentrates by accident). It is also a complication to many other diseases such as mastitis or an infection of the womb (metritis), especially when these diseases occur close to when the goat kids. Spring grass has also been incriminated as a cause of laminitis on account of its high protein content.

Treatment
Whatever the cause of this condition, treatment from your veterinary surgeon is required. Very severe cases may not respond well to treatment, but with modern drugs it is always worth trying. Your veterinary surgeon will most probably prescribe drugs which are anti-inflammatory and relieve the pain in the hoof. In instances where the goat is receiving high quantities of concentrate food, the first step to take, even before you ring the vet, is to reduce the ration.

Prevention
Probably the most important fact to remember is that goats are not really intended to eat concentrate foodstuff. They can do so, but only in relatively limited quantities, and certainly not when it is given suddenly in very large amounts. Remember too, that high-yielding goats, fed maximum quantities of concentrate foodstuff, may in fact be suffering from a very mild form of laminitis. This may pass unnoticed for many months until feet deformities occur and the goats are reluctant to walk. Despite treatment there is a tendency for this condition to recur.

PUNCTURE OF THE SOLE

Dirty objects such as nails or thorns which puncture and penetrate the sole of the hoof, inoculate bacteria into the laminae. If the bacteria multiply in that site pus is produced which soon leads to pain and lameness. Unfortunately the hard horn of the hoof will not allow the pus out, and the goat continues to be lame. This is another job for your veterinary surgeon, who will open the wound, release the pus and also give injections to destroy any germs that have entered. Another possible result of this problem is, of course, tetanus; so always ensure that your goats are protected against this infection by vaccinating them.

WHITE LINE ABSCESS

As described in the introduction to the section on lameness, constant standing in wet faeces and urine can lead to a deterioration of the 'white line'. This is the junction of the wall and the hoof horn, as shown in Figure 3.3. If bacteria penetrate into this space pus forms, causing pain and lameness. Your vet will search out the pus with a hoof knife, relieve the pain and dress the foot.

TREATMENT OF LAME GOATS

Lameness is a symptom of pain somewhere in a limb. It is nature's way of preventing the animal from using that limb and enforcing rest. Although problems can obviously arise anywhere in the limb, in practice most causes of lameness are found in the lower part of the leg, or in the hoof. Always check the upper part of the leg before examining the hoof. It helps to run one's hand down the leg to sense any possible swellings or abnormalities.

Examination of the hoof for unusual signs such as swelling must be carried out. Having established whether or not the lameness arises from the hoof region the goatkeeper must decide whether or not the problem is sufficient to warrant attention from a veterinary surgeon. If your goat has any condition which makes you suspect that the problem arises high up in the limb you should refer the animal to a veterinary surgeon. It is impossible to give strict guidance in respect of foot lameness, but the following indications will hopefully be of value.

Suggested Examination and Treatment that can be Given by the Goatkeeper

- Search for stones or other objects between the claws.
- Trim the hoof.
- Wash the hoof, using a stiff brush (if necessary).
- Examine hoof for penetrating foreign bodies, such as nails.
- Look for signs of infection in the soft tissue between the claws and any evidence of a foul smell.
- Bathe the hoof in copper sulphate or formalin solution; this will rarely do any harm.
- Rest the goat, giving her special attention at feeding time to ensure that the other goats do not bully her.

Problems Requiring Veterinary Attention

- Suspected fractures of the bones.
- Any puncture wound of the hoof, for example where the animal has trodden on a nail.
- Severe lameness, accompanied by an angry red swelling around the top of the hoof (this indicates a sepsis of the foot).
- Any lameness that does not respond to conservative treatment given by the owner over two or three days.
- Any lameness, with blisters around the coronet (*see* FOOT AND MOUTH DISEASE, page 230).
- Goats reluctant to stand, apparently sore on all four feet.
- Any lame goat refusing food.
- Splitting of the horn into the coronet.
- Heat in the hoof.

COCCIDIOSIS

I have included this important problem in this chapter because the condition is most commonly seen in housed goats; indeed housing has a profound effect on its occurrence. It is particularly common in kids above one month of age.

The Coccidia
Agents which are almost always present in the surroundings of goats are the protozoan parasites called coccidia. There are

several stages of this organism's life cycle which take place in the cells of the large and small intestines of the goat. When present in small numbers the coccidia cause very little damage to the goat and no disease. Figure 3.6 illustrates the life cycle of the parasite.

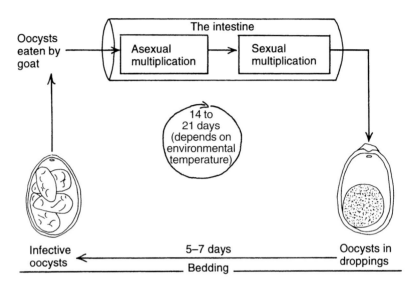

FIGURE 3.6   The life cycle of a coccidium

The number of oocysts (the infective stage of the parasite) put out in the droppings of goats is extremely variable. Does can have counts of between 3,000 and 15,000 oocysts per gram of faeces. Kids with or without signs of disease, can have counts as high as 60,000 oocysts/g. An immune adult goat could put out 216 million oocysts per day and the potential for infecting other goats is obviously very high.

The oocysts in the droppings of one goat become infective to other goats after about one week. (This is very dependent upon temperature.) On ingestion by other goats, they pass through the stomach and into the intestine. The wall of the oocyst breaks down allowing the parasite to invade the lining of the intestine. It is this damage, destruction of cells and the rupturing of blood vessels which give rise to the symptoms of weight loss, diarrhoea or bloody diarrhoea.

Almost all species of animal have their own strain of coccidia and the coccidia of rabbits and chickens, for example, do not cause disease in goats. The coccidia of sheep, however, may be responsible for some disease in goats and therefore should be regarded as suspect. The species of coccidia affecting goats include *Eimeria arloingi, E. faurei, E. christenseni, E. ninakohlyakimovae* and *E. caprovina.*

Symptoms

- *Mild Form*   Kids off their food with symptoms of diarrhoea.
- *Acute Form*   Sick goats with diarrhoea or blood in diarrhoea. The animals are dehydrated and they may show persistent straining in their attempts to pass faeces. Your veterinary surgeon may send samples of the goats' droppings to a laboratory in order to confirm his diagnosis. Goats that recover from coccidiosis may become unthrifty.
- *Very Acute Form*   Recent experimental work suggests that a very acute syndrome can occur resulting in death of the kid within 24 hours. Workers found numerous nodules in the small intestines at post-mortem examination. These were sites of haemorrhagic enteritis. No digestive symptoms were observed. The French workers propose that such nodules may become activated by various stress factors and favour the development of enterotoxaemia.
- Unthrifty kids (chronic effect).

DIAGNOSIS

Clinical signs combined with microscopic examination of the faeces enable us to diagnose coccidiosis. Remember that most goats are infected by coccidia and just demonstrating oocysts in the faeces is not the same as diagnosing the disease of coccidiosis. The laboratory report demonstrating the oocysts should be interpreted by your vet. Some species of coccidia are non-disease causing. In kids, high counts tend to be associated with disease.

Treatment
The first action is to isolate the affected kids to give them better attention as well as to prevent them from further contaminating the pen and spreading the disease to other kids.

Response to drugs given by mouth can be good but treatment must be initiated quickly. Commonly used drugs include sulphonamides and amprolium. Sulphonamides are probably the drug that your veterinary surgeon would prescribe because they have had the dual function of controlling the coccidia and at the same time preventing secondary bacterial infection.

When large numbers of kids are being treated, sulphonamides can be mixed in with the feed or drinking water at a dose rate of 145 mg/kg body weight daily. Amprolium used similarly requires 25 to 50 mg/kg of body weight daily.

When dosing weaned stock, because the kids are often not eating, drinking water administration is the obvious choice. Using tepid water (30° to 35°C) you will have no trouble in getting them to drink. Sulphonamide drugs can cause kidney damage, especially in kids which are dehydrated due to loss of fluids associated with diarrhoea.

Resistance by the coccidia to these treatment compounds has been reported.

Non-specific treatments include the administration of electrolytes instead of milk or milk replacer.

Prevention and control
It is possible to avoid this disease and the answer lies in good management. As a rule of thumb, regard all adults as infected and immune, and all kids as extremely susceptible. The aim of good husbandry is to allow the kids gradual exposure to the agent. This is achieved naturally out at pasture so that the disease is rare when goats are grazing large areas.

Disease is generally seen in housed kids. It can occur in circumstances where they are exposed to infection at a later stage.

Gradual disease-free exposure normally occurs in kids housed in clean pens. The kids experience a small challenge but immunity develops quickly and no disease is seen. Re-infection occurs after ten days and still the kids' developing immunity keeps up with the challenge. The importance of clean and dry bedding cannot be overemphasised. This is especially important as regards areas around drinkers. Avoid overcrowding kids.

There are six situations when disease frequently occurs.

1. When the bedding is very wet and the house is warm and humid. These conditions favour the parasite and allow build-up of oocysts which can overcome the kids' defences.

2. Where pens are not cleaned out between batches of kids. In this instance the first batch of kids grow up with the increasing levels of infection but their increasing immunity matches it. The second batch of young (susceptible) kids soon falls prey to the high levels of challenge, and disease results.

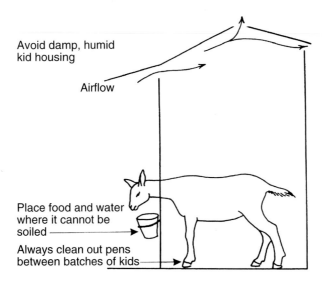

Avoid damp, humid
kid housing

Airflow

Place food and water
where it cannot be
soiled

Always clean out pens
between batches of kids

FIGURE 3.7   The prevention of coccidiosis

3. Where food and water containers become contaminated. Poor design in the siting of food and water containers means that droppings contaminate food and water so that the kids are forced to take in large numbers of oocysts which can result in disease.
4. When susceptible kids are put onto bedding previously used for adult goats.
5. Following stress periods. For example, after a long journey or in the case of angora goats, when penned and weaned.
6. Bought-in goats may introduce new strains of coccidia into the herd. This may even affect adult goats. (See BUYING STOCK page 11.)

The Use of Drugs to Prevent Coccidiosis
Some authors have recommended the use of drugs such as Amprolium to control coccidiosis in groups of kids, where the

problem keeps recurring. Amprolium solution can be added to drinking water or in milk replacer or used as a drench for four to five days. Medication is given for several days every three weeks, the objective being to assist the kids to face a heavy challenge by eliminating the infection while allowing immunity to build up. In my opinion the need for this is extremely rare except, for example, where young goats have to be mixed with older ones. In most cases sensible changes in husbandry would eliminate the need for such medication. I recognise the problems of commercial rearers (20 to 30 kids upwards). I would be the first to admit that when rearing large numbers of kids, coccidiosis is a very difficult problem to avoid. My recommendation would be to put into place the good husbandry practices as described and to keep a sachet of medicine in your cupboard ready for emergencies. Your vet will possibly supply you with a first dose (for use on Sunday evening, for example) and he can reassess the situation the following day.

Coccidiostats
Drugs in this category are given to avoid the problem of coccidiosis in kids. They are administered to healthy goats to prevent a problem occurring. They include Amprolium and Decoquinate.

   None of these compounds are licensed for goats in the UK but they have been used worldwide. If goatkeepers use these coccidiostats advice must be sought from a vet as to withdrawal periods.

The Implications of Coccidiosis
Coccidiosis in replacement kids will have possible repercussions on the next breeding season. Once the intestine of the kid is damaged it takes weeks to recover fully. During that time food absorbtion is reduced, leading to a reduced growth rate. This may prolong the time taken to reach service weight (35 kgs for Saanen kids).

Cleaning and Disinfection
The oocysts (the stage on the bedding) are very resistant to disinfectants and can survive for a year when protected by manure. Sunshine is a valuable aid to destroying the oocysts. When the buildings are emptied after the kids have been reared, try to open up the buildings as much as possible. Expose all the cleaned

feeders and pens to the suns rays in order to reduce the challenge for next years kids.

Worm Control in Yarded and Stall-Fed Goats

Parasites are rarely a problem in adult yarded goats, but it depends upon what is fed to them. The reader should refer to page 111.

SARCOCYSTIS INFECTION

Sarcocystis capracanis is a protozoan parasite of goats. Indian researchers have concluded that sarcocystis infection in conjunction with coccidiosis may increase the severity of coccidiosis.

The disease requires a two-host cycle, for example, dog and goat. In the goat non-specific symptoms such as anorexia, fever and emaciation may occur. A recent report from Iran suggests that no clinical findings were associated with infection of goats by this parasite.

Control of the disease would require separation of the two species but cooking all meat before it is fed to dogs would be beneficial.

Chapter 4

PROBLEMS ASSOCIATED WITH FEEDING

No chapter on this topic would be complete without first of all giving the reader a basic understanding of the anatomy and functioning of the goat's digestive system. The goat belongs to the same family as sheep and cattle, all the members of which are described as 'ruminants'. They are so called because they possess a complex digestive system which incorporates a large stomach or rumen. The function of this organ will be outlined in the text below. Ruminants are therefore very different to simple-stomached (monogastric) animals such as dogs, pigs or humans.

THE ANATOMY OF THE GOAT'S DIGESTIVE SYSTEM

For the sake of clarity this description will commence at the mouth and progress towards the back passage in sequence.

Examination of the mouth of the goat is difficult but the reader should be able to note that unlike humans the goat lacks any incisors or front teeth on the upper jaw. The goat grazes or browses by biting with the front teeth of the lower jaw against a hard pad on the top jaw.

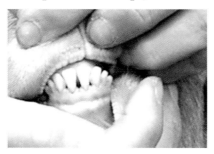 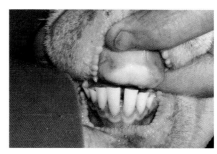

PLATE 4.1 Front teeth – 1 year old   Front teeth – 7 years old

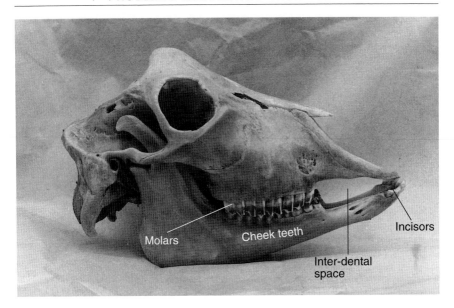

PLATE 4.2 The dentition of a goat, showing an absence of the upper incisors

Assisted by the tongue, the food is then passed back to the cheek teeth where it is given a brief chew before being passed into the oesophagus and on to the stomach. The oesophagus is simply a muscular tube connecting the mouth to the stomach. The stomach is divided into four compartments; listed in the order in which food passes through them they are: (1) rumen, (2) reticulum, (3) omasum and (4) abomasum. Plate 4.3 illustrates their relative size.

Such a digestive apparatus enables ruminants to utilise grass, leaves and other vegetable matter which simple-stomached animals such as a dog are unable to use. After a period of grazing or browsing the goat commences to ruminate or 'chew the cud'. This involves moving food material back up the oesophagus to the mouth where it is chewed between the goat's back teeth. Following this chewing, the food is returned to the rumen where it remains for several hours undergoing fermentation. Gas is produced as a result of this fermentation and this must be eliminated by the goat belching frequently.

It is during this fermentation process that nutrients are unlocked from the vegetable matter of the goat's diet. The contents of the cells of plants are not available to most monogastric

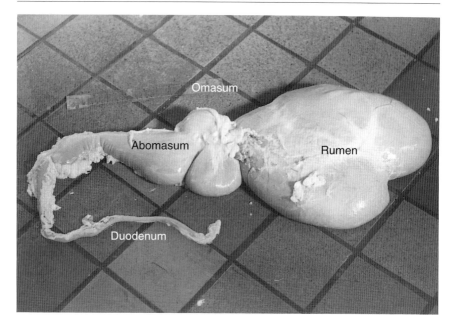

PLATE 4.3   Stomach and duodenum of an adult goat

animals because they lack the enzymes necessary to digest the plant cell wall. Goats also lack these enzymes but they solve the problem by allowing bacteria and micro-organisms to do the job for them. Goats provide the bacteria with a suitable warm place to live: the rumen, and in return the bacteria release, for the goat's benefit, the food locked up in the plant cells. Some vitamins are also made available for the goat. After the food has been fermented in the rumen and reticulum it gradually passes through the omasum or 'bible', where further grinding of the food particles takes place.

From here it passes into the abomasum or true stomach, an organ not dissimilar to our own. Digestive enzymes mix with the food in the abomasum and this muscular sack pushes food through into the small intestine at regular intervals.

In the small intestine further digestive juices are secreted along with those from the liver and pancreas. A great deal of absorption of nutrients occurs in this part of the digestive tract.

The caecum, situated at the beginning of the large intestine, is a blind-ending sack in which some absorption of fluids takes place. The large intestine functions mainly to resorb water from the products of digestion which pass through it. The familiar 'pellets' of the goat form in the last part of the large bowel or colon, and from here pass out through the rectum.

There are several important comments one can make at this stage in relation to this digestive system.

- The goat must always be able to get rid of the gas formed in the rumen otherwise bloat develops (*see* BLOAT, page 139).
- The rumen is a large fermentation chamber, full of many beneficial micro-organisms which live in delicate balance.
- The capacity of the rumen is great: two gallons in the adult goat. Should a goat gain access to concentrate foodstuffs by mistake she can consume vast quantities, more than is good for her.
- Adult goats vomit with difficulty, and therefore anything taken into the rumen by mistake is well and truly locked within the animal.

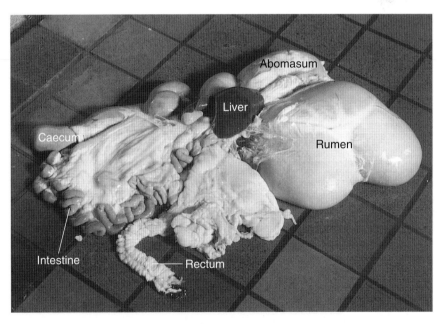

PLATE 4.4   Stomach and intestines of an adult goat

Kids

The diet of kids is of course milk, and the complex stomach of the adult animal is not required. Up to about six weeks of age only the abomasum or 'true stomach' is working and the kid's digestive system functions rather like that of the monogastric animal (*see* page 23).

Teeth and Problems of Sore Mouths

Goats may refuse food for two basic reasons. Firstly they may feel ill and disinclined to eat and secondly they may find the eating process painful. Typical reasons for the latter are painful teeth or injuries to the soft tissues of the mouth. Goats with mild pain in the mouth may just eat very slowly or drop food from the mouth. They may drool saliva and 'smack' their lips. In such instances the goatkeeper should examine the mouth in order to try and determine the cause.

Unfortunately it is very difficult to open the mouths of goats in order to make such an examination, and it may be necessary to sedate the goat. Remember not to place your fingers between the back teeth as this can result in a painful injury. Swellings of the soft tissue of the mouth frequently result from small injuries which sometimes become serious enough to warrant a course of antibiotic injections.

'Choke', Oesophageal Obstruction

Occasionally goats suffer from choke when an object of food material obstructs the oesophagus, preventing belching. This is a potentially dangerous situation because the build-up of gas in the rumen can very quickly cause death (*see* Bloat page 139).

Action to be taken in the event of choke
Call your vet who will probably try to relax the oesophagus using a smooth muscle-relaxant; he may pass a stomach tube in order to dislodge the obstruction. If this action fails he may be obliged to perform a small operation in order to remove the offending object. This is done by cutting into the oesophagus from outside. (*See* also page 259.)

Bloat
See Chapter 5, 'Problems Associated with Grazing', page 139.

INDIGESTION

Occasionally goats in peak lactation may suffer from indigestion resulting in loss of appetite. There is failure of the normal rumenal movement and cudding ceases. It is usually associated with high intake of concentrate foodstuffs. Many mild diseases may cause indigestion but are of little significance.

Symptoms
The goat is off its food, slightly dull and suffers a small fall in milk yield. There are few other signs, and generally the goat recovers within two days.

Treatment
Generally this is not essential but mild rumenal stimulants may help. Sodium bicarbonate given by mouth may be of some use if there is a tendency to acid conditions in the rumen. Offer the goat two litres of tepid water with 25 g of sodium bicarbonate and 10 g of table salt dissolved in it.

ACIDOSIS

This is the term given to the condition when the rumen contents become acid. It can be described as acute or chronic. Acute acidosis generally occurs after a goat has accidentally taken in large quantities of concentrate foodstuffs when, for example, the store shed has been left open by mistake and the goatkeeper finds the goats eating buckets of dairy cubes. This is probably one of the most serious accidents that can befall a goat. The rumen becomes full of concentrates which quickly ferment to acid (pH 5 or less). The acid is absorbed from the rumen into the bloodstream causing the animal to feel ill and damaging its metabolism.

An important factor in this disease is the previous diet of the goat involved. A heavy milker that is receiving over a kilogram of concentrate may be relatively unaffected by this quantity, because her rumen is adapted to it. On the other hand, a goat at pasture which suddenly consumes that quantity of feed may become extremely ill. The types of foodstuff that give rise to easily fermentable substrate include sugar beet, dairy cubes and all the cereal grains.

Symptoms
These can vary depending upon the previous diet of the goat and on the quantity of food consumed. In the early stages the goat becomes depressed and hangs its head. Later the goat becomes intoxicated and 'drunken' in behaviour; muscle twitching may be observed. Bloat tends to occur and there is a swelling on the left flank (*see* page 140). Because of the pain the goat may grind its teeth and diarrhoea soon becomes apparent. Eventually the goat 'goes down' and is unable to rise, a truly sorry state. Very acute cases die within 24 hours. Cases that survive tend to become lame as a result of laminitis. Recent studies also revealed liver damage to be an important sequel.

Treatment
This condition must be treated as an emergency by the goat-keeper. Veterinary attention must be sought if the animal is to have a chance of survival. The first thing to do is of course to stop access to any more food. A first-aid measure would be to drench the goat with something alkaline such as bicarbonate of soda (or baking powder). Two or three ounces (50 g) will help neutralise the acid. Walking the goat up and down is probably of some value as well.

Your veterinary surgeon may decide upon a number of different treatments, depending upon the case. He may choose to operate on the goat in order to remove the foodstuff directly from the rumen. He will probably only do this if the goat is still in reasonable shape because dehydration occurs, making the animal a poor surgical risk. One report described the transfer of rumen contents from healthy cows to make up for the acid rumen content removed. Many cases are treated by drugs alone; yeasts may be useful by mouth. Fluids obviously help in dehydrated cases: intravenous drips of isotonic sodium chloride and 5 per cent sodium bicarbonate solution. Vitamin injections can help to detoxify the animal. Sometimes antihistamine drugs are given to overcome laminitis, which can result from acidosis. NSAID compounds could also be helpful.

Diagnosis
The recent history of the animal will be important for your vet, for example, that the goat had access to too much maize or beet pulp. He may then proceed to take a sample of rumen fluid, using a needle directly into the rumen and withdrawing 5 to 10 ml in a syringe. The pH test can be carried out on this fluid.

Chronic acidosis is seen in intensively kept goats (*see* ACIDOSIS AND THE MILKER'S RATION). It is slower in onset, characterised by a fall in milk production, slowing down of rumination and picky appetite.

ACIDOSIS AND THE MILKER'S RATION

Not infrequently, high yielding dairy goats can become acidotic as a result of being fed large quantities of concentrate food. Some guidelines may be useful in this context. The problems tend to arise when changes are made to the ration to adjust for increasing milk yield in early lactation. The following simple rules may help you to avoid the problem.

- Make any feed changes gradually over several days to allow the rumen micro-organisms time to adjust.
- Distribute the concentrate portion of the ration in several small meals a day, i.e. four times a day rather than at each milking.
- Feed at least half the total ration, in terms of dry matter, as long fibre foods (hay, grass, silage, etc).
- Keep stressful changes to a minimum (mixing animals, change of routine, etc).
- Always keep some sodium bicarbonate to hand. Never be afraid to offer a sick goat 25 g of sodium bicarbonate in a litre of tepid water, if you feel she has taken in too much concentrate.

ALKALOSIS

The opposite condition to acidosis (above) arises when there is a tendency for the rumen pH to be alkaline. The alkaline pH reduces the growth of rumen micro-organisms. Generally this occurs when there is an excess of ammonia in the rumen resulting from an excess of protein in the diet or a relative lack of carbohydrate in the ration. The condition might appear in goats turned out onto lush spring grass.

Symptoms
Muddy soft black faeces, slightly distended abdomens, possibly goats with nervous symptoms.

Action to take

Correct the ration by reducing the total protein and if necessary adjusting the carbohydrate balance. Dosing the goats with a little vinegar in water may help to reduce the alkaline pH of the rumen.

DISPLACEMENT OF THE ABOMASUM

Very, very rarely, a condition occurs when the fourth stomach moves from the right-hand side of the abdomen to the left-hand side. It becomes trapped between the rumen and the left flank wall, giving rise to a specific syndrome.

The Reason for Displacement

The condition is thought to occur just after kidding. During pregnancy the uterus expands, pushing the abomasum under the rumen. The rumen also tends to rise as a result of this pressure. It is believed that after kidding the rumen falls down, trapping the abomasum.

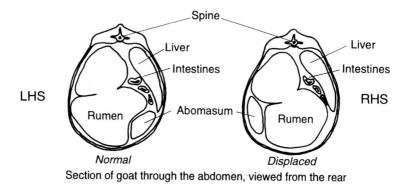

Section of goat through the abdomen, viewed from the rear

FIGURE 4.1   Normal and displaced positions of the abomasum

Symptoms

The condition is noted to occur around parturition (kidding). The appetite of affected goats becomes reduced; they tend to pick at their food and refuse concentrates. Milk yield would obviously be reduced. Your veterinary surgeon will confirm his suspicion by listening to characteristic sounds on the left flank.

Treatment
In cattle, where the disease is relatively common, two forms of treatment are used; one involves surgery, the other does not.

- *Surgical repair* The surgeon pulls back the fourth stomach and stitches it to the right-hand flank wall.
- *Rolling* In cattle, rolling the animal on its back in the correct manner can restore the stomach to its former position. I have a suspicion that some cases resolve themselves during the journey by car to the vet's surgery. On more than one occasion symptoms of this condition have been described to me on the telephone but the goat appears 'cured' when she arrives!

Prevention
There are precious few records of this condition in goats so one must look to work in cattle for some guidance. One may postulate that avoiding heavy concentrate feeding during pregnancy may help to avoid the problem occurring. The main reason for this is that heavy concentrate feed will result in a small rumen (less bulk) and therefore allow the displacement to occur more easily. Feed good quality fibre (good hay). I must stress again, that this is a rare condition in goats.

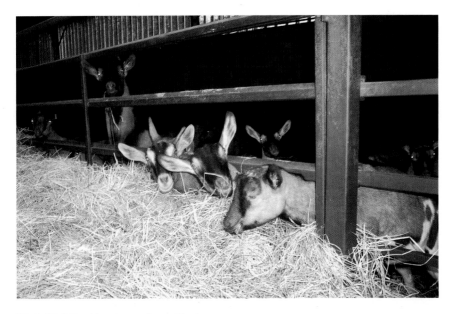

PLATE 4.5   Feed good quality forage

Aflatoxicosis (Mould Poisoning)

Foodstuffs such as groundnuts, soya beans and cereals some-times become contaminated by fungus or mould. The toxins damage the liver, reducing its efficiency. Symptoms include loss of condition, reduced appetite and possibly jaundice. In an incident in Sri Lanka, 194 out of 1800 kids died. They were mainly aged between 6 and 9 months, and at post-mortem exam-ination the livers were found to be destroyed, being hard and fibrous. This problem is thankfully rare in developed countries with good laboratory facilities.

Treatment
In mild cases vitamins and supportive therapy may help the animal survive and some liver regeneration takes place.

Pregnancy Toxaemia

This is a metabolic disease of does in late pregnancy. It is non-infectious, being a product of disturbed carbohydrate usage. It can be caused by either faulty feeding or starvation.

Figure 4.2 shows the normal situation for a non-pregnant, non-lactating doe. She represents an animal with the least demand for nutrients because all she requires is enough to main-tain her tissues in working order.

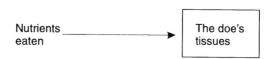

FIGURE 4.2   *The energy requirements (maintenance) of a non-producing doe*

A goat in late pregnancy obviously has extra demand upon the supply of food especially for carbohydrate (energy) foods, as shown in Figure 4.3.

If in fact the doe is carrying twins or triplets, then the burden may be too high unless the food contains a large amount of energy. Some foods – for example, poor-quality hay – may have

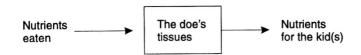

FIGURE 4.3 The energy requirements (maintenance and production) of a
pregnant doe

enough energy for a non-pregnant goat, but insufficient amounts
for a doe carrying twins. Also, in late pregnancy the uterus and
its contents take up a large amount of space in the doe's abdomen
so that she cannot possibly eat enough poor-quality foodstuff to
provide all her requirements. (*See* Figure 4.4.)

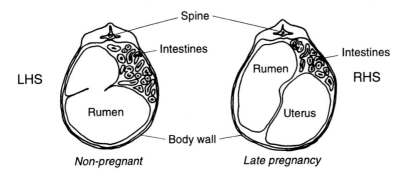

FIGURE 4.4 Effect of the uterus on the rumen of a heavily pregnant doe

When this state of affairs occurs the doe ensures that the kids
get enough carbohydrates at the expense of her own tissues. She
then robs her own reserves of carbohydrates and this leads to the
release of ketone bodies into her blood – a sign that her metabolism is faulty. Paradoxically, the condition is also seen in
over-fat does that have been allowed to gain too much weight in
early pregnancy.

Symptoms
Lethargy and loss of appetite over one to two weeks, generally in
very late pregnancy (about 140 days). Cases tend to become
recumbent and have sweet-smelling (ketotic) breath. Grinding of
the teeth and moaning are commonly observed. If untreated, convulsions may occur, and the goat will die within a week. This is

an extremely serious condition and treatment should be initiated as soon as possible.

Treatment

Response to treatment is not very good, although it is well worth attempting it. There are two basic objectives: (1) to give the doe a readily usable form of energy such as glucose; (2) to get her eating again (using anabolic steroids such as trenbolone acetate).

Of course she still has kids inside draining away any energy you give her and so many vets either encourage the doe to deliver her kids early (alive or dead), or perform a caesarean section. The decision depends upon the value of the kids, the stage of the pregnancy and the condition of the doe.

As a first-aid treatment, before the vet arrives, the owner could drench the goat with glucose in water or molasses (treacle) in water; 100 g of either would do some good.

Prevention

- Slim down fat goats before mating.
- Feed good-quality forage in the last two months of pregnancy.
- Daily exercise may be useful.
- Ensure palatable food is offered in late pregnancy.
- Scan the goats to determine the number of kids in the uterus.
- Always supplement forage in the last six weeks of pregnancy with some concentrate (in case the goat is carrying twins or triplets). Remember that three-quarters of goat pregnancies result in the birth of two or more kids. The nutrient requirements for a pregnant goat weighing 70 kg two months before kidding are:

Dry matter kg/day 1.5   *ME MJ/day* 15.5   *DCP g/day* 121.

This means that the doe should eat 15.5 mega joules (ME) of energy food plus 121 g of digestible crude protein (DCP) contained in 1.5 kg of dry matter (DM). For example, if 1.2 kg of hay is fed and this contains 1 kg of dry matter (DM) which provides 11 mega joules of metabolisable energy (ME), then the goat should receive a further 4.5 MJ of energy in its concentrate ration contained in perhaps 0.6 kg of concentrate (0.5 kg DM of concentrate). For further explanation the reader should refer to a textbook on nutrition such as:

- Agricultural Research Council (1984) *The Nutrient Requirements of Ruminant Livestock Supplement, No. 1.* Commonwealth Agricultural Bureaux, Farnham Royal, Bucks.
- Orskov, E. R. (1987) *The Feeding of Ruminants: Principles and Practice.* Chalcombe Publications, 18 Sudbeck Lane, Welton Lincoln, LN2 3JF, UK

Notes for Veterinarians
Betamethasone, PGF2 alpha or a combination of both have been successfully used to induce labour. Parturition results 6–36 hours later.

Dosage guide:
  Lutalase (Pfizer)) 1 ml
  Estrumate (Schering-Plough) 0.5 ml
  Betsolan (Schering-Plough) 3 to 4 ml

ACETONAEMIA (KETOSIS)

This condition is remarkably similar to pregnancy toxaemia described in the last section. The main difference is the time when acetonaemia manifests itself, being characteristically in the first month of lactation. Another feature is that it is a disease of housed does in the winter months.

Why the Disease Occurs
Referring back to Figures 4.2 and 4.3, the lactating doe is similar to the pregnant doe in terms of requirement for carbohydrate because a great deal is required for milk production. This could be represented as Figure 4.5.

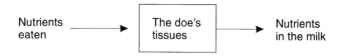

FIGURE 4.5 *The energy requirements (maintenance and production) of a lactating doe*

Obviously the high-yielding doe in peak lactation (about 4 weeks after kidding), requires enormous amounts of energy feed.

If she is unable to obtain this, the same circumstances prevail as in pregnancy toxaemia. Ketones (acetones) accumulate in the blood and this is described as acetonaemia.

Symptoms
The doe goes off her food, tending to prefer hay to concentrates. Milk yield falls and the goatkeeper may be able to detect a sweet smell in the goat's breath (this is the smell of the acetone).

Treatment
This is theoretically more simple than treating pregnancy toxaemia and the condition can respond to treatment very quickly. On the other hand many stubborn protracted recoveries have been widely reported. Treatment can often be to no avail. Again, as a first-aid treatment, a glucose or treacle drench may be given. Your veterinary surgeon may inject the goat with a corticosteroid drug which usually dramatically reverses the condition. An intravenous injection of glucose (dextrose) is also necessary (40 ml of a 50 per cent solution). The vet may prescribe easily used, high-energy substances, such as propylene glycol to be given by mouth. Multivitamin injections may also be of value. Once the goat has regained her appetite increase her ration of energy food (cereals) so that a relapse does not occur.

Prevention
As with pregnancy toxaemia, ensure does are lean before mating and keep them from getting fat in early pregnancy. After kidding aim at ensuring adequate levels of concentrates for high-yielders. It may be necessary to feed concentrate little and often because the doe finds it difficult to eat enough to keep up with the tremendous output of milk. You can help by giving the goat daily exercise and possibly by feeding titbits of green foods to stimulate appetite. You may learn a great deal about this condition by discussing feeding with a local dairy cow farmer. The principles are the same for dairy cows and goats.

DIETARY SCOUR (DIARRHOEA) IN ADULT GOATS

Occasionally, changes in diet result in diarrhoea in the adult goat. Every animal has a population of micro-organisms in the gut which in normal circumstances live in a stable situation. Following a change in the type of food eaten certain bacteria begin to multiply and take over, because the conditions become just right for them. Such a situation can result in toxins irritating the gut lining, causing massive outpourings of fluids. Absorption of food declines and diarrhoea results. Dietary scour is quite commonly diagnosed in veterinary practice.

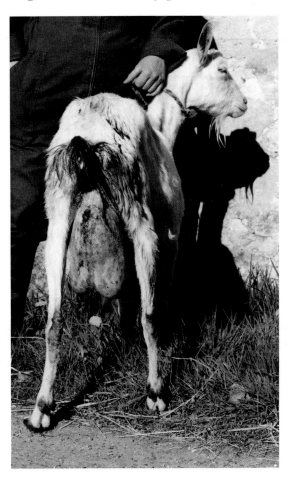

PLATE 4.6   Diarrhoea

The Danger of Enterotoxaemia
Such circumstances, i.e. diarrhoea, are ideal for the development of enterotoxaemia. The conditions allow the multiplication of certain clostridial bacteria. Remember to have all goats vaccinated against this.

Symptoms

Generally, uncomplicated dietary scour gives rise to few other symptoms, although there may be a fall in milk yield in lactating animals.

Treatment

Cutting food back is important, especially restricting the quantity of the new type of food material. In many cases this action alone will restore the goat to normality. Hay is a very useful feed for goats suffering from diarrhoea; oak leaves help, but have a constipatory action.

The standard treatment should be to give the goat a proprietary electrolyte powder such as Lectade (Pfizer Limited), dissolved in tepid water. Offer the goat the contents of the packet, made-up as directed. If you do not have such a proprietary treatment administer one dessertspoonful (50 g) of glucose plus one teaspoonful (10 g) of table salt in 1.5 litres of tepid water, offered in a bucket.

In more severe cases all sorts of remedies are available including kaolin. Antibiotics should not be necessary but your vet may give the goat an injection of drugs such as Buscopan compositum (each ml contains 4 mg butylscopolamine bromide and 500 mg metamizole (INN) as active ingredients plus 5 mg of phenol as preservative) which slows down the passage of fluids through the intestine.

Prevention

It seems very obvious, but it never does any harm to stress the need to introduce new dietary compounds slowly. This allows the micro-organisms in the gut to adapt gradually to the new food.

INTESTINAL OBSTRUCTION (BLOCKAGE)

This is fortunately a rare event in the goat, which I have never seen, but I shall describe it for the sake of completeness. It could result from many causes such as a telescoping effect of the bowel (called an intussusception) or, possibly, adhesions. One case was caused by a plastic bag. The symptoms would be those of a sick goat which has no appetite, possibly a distended abdomen and is passing no droppings. Because of the pain, teeth-grinding and belly-kicking might be noted. The early signs may be restricted to paleness of the mucous membranes (inside the mouth, around the eye, the vagina) and a sub-normal temperature. The outcome can often be fatal. To examine the mucous membranes look inside the mouth or vaginal lips or turn down the eyelid (*see* plate 5.2, page 108).

Cerebro Cortical Necrosis (CCN)

At first sight it may seem strange to include a condition of brain malfunction in this chapter on feeding but the two are related. This condition, occurring in goats of any age but predominant in the young, gives rise to nervous symptoms. The symptoms result from necrosis or death of some of the cells in the cortex of the brain. The explanation for the death of these cells is a lack of thiamine (vitamin B_1).

Thiamine is normally present in adequate quantities in the rumen. In certain circumstances, however, the rumen flora change to favour a population of organisms that produce thiaminase. This enzyme destroys the thiamine and causes a deficiency. The brain has a high demand for thiamine and problems are manifested by various nervous symptoms. Acidotic rumen conditions (high concentrate feeding) are probably very significant as a cause of this condition in intensively kept goats.

Symptoms
The goat shows nervous symptoms such as blindness, trembling, rigidity and also standing with the head pressed against a wall. They may wander in circles and even develop convulsions. These symptoms are similar to those of other diseases such as lead poisoning so your veterinary surgeon will probably send samples to a laboratory for diagnosis.

Treatment
The administration of thiamine is obviously useful but the response to treatment may be poor if the brain is too badly damaged. In cases treated early, a rapid response can be seen within two hours.

The dose of thiamine is 500 mg for a kid weighing 20 kg and 1 g for an adult goat, preferably half of the dose being given intravenously. French workers suggest frequent (every six hours) intravenous doses of 10 mg/Kg for the first 24 hours. The other goats in the group should have their concentrate ration reduced. Sodium bicarbonate at 10 g per goat can usefully be given to all the animals in order to reduce the chance of acidosis developing.

Vitamin B₁ (thiamine) can be fed at 150 mg daily for 10 days.

One report from the United States declared that only three out of six treated goats responded to thiamine therapy. The other three died between two and seven days after the onset of symptoms. All the goats were being fed concentrates and the outbreak occurred during the winter.

LISTERIOSIS

Goats fed on silage are prone to develop symptoms of listeriosis, an infection caused by Listeria monocytogenes. The conditions produced when making silage are often conducive to the proliferation of the organism. (*See* LISTERIOSIS, page 233)

DEFICIENCIES OF ESSENTIAL DIETARY COMPONENTS (VITAMINS AND MINERALS)

VITAMINS

The vitamins are a group of compounds that have been shown to be essential for the normal functioning of the goat and other animals. They are only required in very small quantities but if they are absent from the diet the effect can be quite dramatic.

Unlike monogastric animals, goats are able to manufacture some of their vitamins, or at least the rumen micro-organisms do it for them. Vitamin D can of course be produced by the skin in the presence of sunlight. The stress laid upon vitamin deficiencies by the manufacturers of vitamin products is probably over-emphasised. That does not mean to say that goatkeepers should not be aware of possible deficiency states.

The Diet and Vitamin Supply

Vitamins are present in varying quantities in different food substances. It is fairly obvious, therefore, that a goat fed a varied diet is more likely to avoid the pitfalls of vitamin deficiency than is a goat whose diet is more restricted. By feeding a little of this substance and a little of that, deficiencies can normally be avoided, even if the goatkeeper is unaware of the specific components of each kind of foodstuff.

Goatkeepers with small herds easily achieve a variety of

foodstuffs by feeding browse, allowing access to grazing and perhaps some concentrates.

Vitamins and Stress and Disease

Bacterial infections increase the demand for some vitamins such as vitamin A. When animals are ill they are generally off their food and hence, in sickness, goats may benefit from extra vitamins. Stress conditions are also thought to increase the requirement for vitamins.

VITAMIN A

This vitamin is essential for the health of all the lining surfaces of the goat's body; for example, the skin and the cells lining the gut. It is taken in by the grazing goat in the form of protovitamin A and is converted into vitamin A mainly by the intestinal wall. Good pasture contains adequate quantities (between 3 and 8 mg per cent) and fresh hay less, between 1 and 2 mg per cent. Reserves can be stored in the liver for a few months. Calves born to cows grazed on pasture have higher levels than calves born to stable-kept cows. This is probably true of goats and their kids.

Symptoms of deficiency
Because this vitamin is essential for the lining surfaces, a lack of it can cause deficiencies of any of these surfaces (the gut, windpipe and bronchi, urinary tract etc). Thus diarrhoea and respiratory disease will be likely. Blindness may also occur. In one recorded problem in a herd of 223 goats the following symptoms predominated: abortion, diarrhoea and the loss of sight due to the opacity of the cornea. The problem is likely to occur only on very poor pasture or when yarded goats are fed very poor diets for long periods.

Treatment
Response to treatment with vitamin A is generally good. Toxicity resulting from too much vitamin A has occasionally been recorded but it is most unlikely to occur unless doses of 200 times the normal level are given over long periods. A suitable time for dosing is late pregnancy, which will benefit both the dam and the kid.

VITAMIN D

This vitamin regulates the calcium and phosphorus in the animal's body. It acts in several ways, which include increasing the mineralisation of bones and teeth. It is present in green foods but low in stored hay. Animals can manufacture their own vitamin D in the skin, in the presence of sunlight.

Symptoms
Poor growth and feed conversion. The disease is termed rickets in the young and osteomalacia, or bone softening, in the adult. Osteomalacia is very rare but gives symptoms of stiffness and crippling. (*See* also page 100.)

RICKETS

Rickets can occur in young rapidly growing goat kids, although it is uncommon in Europe and North America. It can result from a deficiency of either calcium or phosphorus or vitamin D. When any one of these factors is missing from the diet defective bone formation occurs.

Symptoms
Stiffness of movement characterises this condition, accompanied by enlarged joints, especially of the front legs. It may also be possible to feel a swelling half way down each rib, forming a chain along the chest. The joint swelling results from poorly mineralised bone undergoing pressure and becoming deformed.

Treatment
Providing a balanced diet containing calcium and phosphorus is the key to success. Exposing the animals to sunlight enables them to manufacture their own vitamin D in the skin. Injections of vitamin D may be given by your vet.

Prevention
As stressed under Treatment, a well-balanced diet, containing minerals, is essential. If one is ever concerned about possible deficiencies in feedstuffs remember that by ensuring variety in the diet one often avoids deficiency.

Vitamin E and White Muscle Disease

Vitamin E is present in hay and grass and to a lesser degree in cereals. Deficiency is only likely to occur in animals kept on poor-quality rations. The activities of this vitamin are poorly understood, though it is considered to act as an antioxidant. Its functions are closely bound up with the mineral selenium: in some circumstances either selenium or vitamin E will prevent problems. Soils and pastures vary widely in their content of selenium.

Symptoms
A deficiency of this vitamin disturbs both cell metabolism and the structure of all the component living parts of the cell. The principal symptoms of deficiency are associated with muscles, that is, the degeneration of heart and skeletal muscle. The muscle fibres become pale and hence the name 'white muscle'. Stress and disease conditions are thought to increase the requirements for vitamin E.

Two types of symptom are described: mild and acute. In the mild form stiffness, weakness and trembling are reported. In the acute form affected animals are found dead without showing any previous signs. Thus, most of our knowledge of the disease comes from work on dead animals, at post-mortem examinations. When examined, all the evidence of muscle damage can be seen in the heart, diaphragm and legs. White streaks of unhealthy tissue can be seen among the normal muscle fibres. Unfortunately tests for the deficiency are not useful on a routine basis and most goatkeepers only learn of problems after deaths have occurred. Emphasis must therefore be placed on prevention of the disease.

Treatment
Normally the administration of selenium, together with vitamin E, will reverse the symptoms within a week. Vitamin E preparations can be given either by mouth or injection.

Prevention
A varied diet with a plentiful supply of good-quality hay, made while the plant is still green, will normally ensure freedom from the disease. The condition is extremely unlikely to occur while animals are at pasture. Yarded animals, fed on diets such as roots

(known to be low in vitamin E), should receive supplementation in their diet. Add, for example, sodium selenite. Otherwise, an injectable preparation of selenium should be given (e.g. Vitenium [Novartis]). Discuss this with your vet. Do not over-dose, otherwise selenium poisoning may result.

Vitamins C and K

Both these vitamins are present in grass and hay. They can also be manufactured by the bacteria in the rumen (vitamin K) or in the liver and kidneys (vitamin C). Deficiencies of these vitamins, therefore, do not occur and no extra supplements need be given. Where goats have had access to Warfarin-type rat poisons, then an induced deficiency may result.

Minerals and Diet

Minerals such as calcium and phosphorus are essential as com-ponents of bone and teeth. They are required in large amounts, especially in the growing kid, which is rapidly building up bone tissue.

Trace Elements
Some minerals are only required in minute quantities and, as only a trace is needed for healthy functioning, they are described as 'trace elements'. Manganese and copper are examples of these elements.

The Turnover of Minerals
The complement of minerals within the goat's body is never static but is continuously changing. Minerals are continually being taken in along with the food and simultaneously lost from the body. In order to remain healthy, however, the delicate balance must be maintained and very complex regulation takes place. This regulation is sometimes carried out by hormones such as the parathyroid hormone. An important fact to note is that minerals must always be available for use by the goat. It is no use giving large quantities at intervals and then depriving the goat for weeks.

Mineral Deficiencies
In well-managed goats, fed a variety of foodstuffs, deficiencies are very unusual. Well-documented laboratory experiments have been conducted so that scientists do know the effects of deficiency of numerous minerals but in the field these are extremely rare. Feeding imbalances occur from time to time and some of them are dealt with in the following section. In such instances, errors often arise as a result of feeding one nutrient in quantities which influence another nutrient. Many goatkeepers buy proprietary mineral supplements or provide ad-lib access to lick blocks, which allow the goats to supplement those in the food. Discuss these products with your local feed supplier.

COBALT DEFICIENCY

Cobalt is essential for the production of vitamin B_{12} by micro-organisms in the rumen. Deficiency leads to a wasting condition in sheep and goats called 'pine' which has rather vague symptoms. The lack of vitamin B_{12} (cyanocobalamin) leads to loss of appetite, and thus affected goats simply do not eat and they waste away.

Symptoms
Loss of body weight, poor appetite and anaemia are classic symptoms. This condition may be compounded by worms because the deficiency makes goats more susceptible to roundworm parasites. The animals can literally pine away and die.

Treatment
Cobalt can be given by mouth, or vitamin B_{12} may be given by injection. 'Bullets' containing cobalt are available but they are only of use in kids over two to three months of age. These allow the slow release of cobalt into the rumen.

Prevention
The use of cobalt bullets is the most convenient method of preventing this disease in deficient areas. Also, provide proprietary lick-blocks containing cobalt. Areas of the world affected by cobalt deficiency are well known to veterinary surgeons so your vet will probably guide you on this. (*See also* PINE, page 138.) Some wormers incorporate cobalt to help avoid deficiencies.

COPPER DEFICIENCY

The effects of copper deficiency on pregnant does result in their giving birth to kids with swayback (*see* ENZOOTIC ATAXIA, page 46).

In cattle and sheep, deficiency of copper also gives rise to a variety of symptoms such as anaemia, poor growth and loss of milk production. Similar symptoms can occur in goats. Low blood copper levels (hypocupraemia) are sometimes demonstrated by laboratory tests.

It may be important to note that another mineral, molybdenum, has an action directly opposite to that of copper and therefore copper deficiency has been recorded in areas where soil molybdenum levels are high.

Treatment and prevention

If copper deficiency is confirmed goats can be given copper either by injection or dosing by mouth. One method is to administer copper oxide needles by oral dosing. These fragments (below 8 mm) are retained in the forestomachs for up to 100 days. Copper is very toxic, however, and guidance should be obtained from your veterinary surgeon on how much to give. Provide proprietary lick-blocks containing copper.

Copper Poisoning

The metabolism of copper in the goat appears to be different from that in sheep. Goats are in fact more resistant to copper poisoning than sheep because less copper accumulates in the liver.

The mechanism of copper poisoning is complex but involves a haemolytic crisis when red blood cells are destroyed, leading to fatal complications in the body. Situations where poisoning can occur include dietary excess from incorrect supplementation and grazing pastures after pig manure has been recently spread.

Symptoms include lack of appetite, dullness and blood-stained urine. The animals may simply be found dead.

IODINE DEFICIENCY

Occasionally this element can be deficient in the diet, giving rise to 'goitre' or swollen thyroid glands. It may also be induced because the animals are consuming goitrogenic (goitre producing) foods such as kale. Goitrogenic substances lock up the iodine in the food and cause a deficiency. Iodine is essential for the production of thyroid hormone, an important body regulator which has a profound effect upon the rate of the body's chemical reactions.

Symptoms
These are most obvious in newborn kids which show weakness, absence of hair and large thyroid glands. They can also be seen in fast-growing kids because milk is a poor source of iodine. The thyroid glands may also be enlarged in adult goats. A recent report from Italy describes a case in which half of the winter born kids were lost from hypothyroid goitre.

Treatment and prevention
This condition is reversible and it is always worth attempting to treat affected animals. Because of the toxicity of iodine, treatment doses should be as little as doses aimed at prevention. Feeding iodised salt (containing at least 0.007 per cent iodine) is one method of prevention. Alternatively potassium iodide can be given by mouth or solution of iodine can be applied to the animal's coat once a week. This will be licked off by the goat. For oral administration, 2 ml of a 2 per cent solution of iodine in potassium iodide gives good results.

SALT (SODIUM CHLORIDE) DEFICIENCY

Sodium and chlorine are essential for maintenance of the tissue fluids and they are vital for numerous bodily conditions such as nerve transmission and water balance. I know of no specific deficiency reports in goats, but in heavily lactating dairy cows deficiency is thought to be widespread. Proprietary concentrate rations, such as dairy cubes, contain 1 per cent sodium chloride.

Prevention
Give goats access to salt in the form of a lick or loose crystals, especially when they are lactating and at pasture.

ZINC DEFICIENCY

This condition has been produced experimentally in goats; the symptoms were those of a thickened skin. Dietary supplementation would reverse the condition should it occur naturally. Recently the problem was diagnosed in goats showing loss of hair and skin thickening. Abnormalities of the feet were also described. The zinc levels in the serum were 0.64 mg/ml and 0.55 mg/ml. The symptoms rapidly disappeared when treatment with 250 mg of zinc sulphate was given by mouth.

SELENIUM DEFICIENCY

The effects of deficiency of selenium are to produce muscular dystrophy. There is an intimate relationship between vitamin E and selenium; either substance will reverse a deficiency state of the other (*see* VITAMIN E, page 95). Some wormers incorporate selenium to help prevent deficiencies in small ruminants.

Selenium Toxicity
A toxicity from excess selenium can occur from eating herbage containing high levels of selenium but this is very rare and has only been reported in Ireland. In the acute form, nervous symptoms are noted and in the chronic form, lameness and weight loss are reported.

DISEASES ASSOCIATED WITH DEFICIENCY AND IMBALANCE OF PHOSPHORUS, CALCIUM AND VITAMIN D

A disturbance of intake or metabolism of either of these two minerals tends to be very complex. There is also the inter-relationship between them and vitamin D. Deficiencies of vitamin D have been covered on page 94. Sometimes enough calcium and phosphorus are fed in adequate quantities but they are fed in the wrong proportions. The suggested calcium to phosphorus ratio is between 2:1 and 1:1 calcium to phosphorus. Large amounts of calcium are present in the teeth and bones. Disturbances show up in the teeth and bones when they are fed incorrectly.

Sources of Calcium and Phosphorus

Calcium is normally present in the leafy parts of plants where phosphorus is relatively low. Phosphorus is found in relatively high levels in cereal grains. Calcium is normally added to the proprietary concentrate rations sold for feeding to lactating dairy animals.

OSTEODYSTROPHIA FIBROSA

This condition is caused by feeding too high a ratio of phosphorus to calcium. It results in a decalcification of the bones, particularly of the skull. Growing animals are most seriously affected. It is rare in goats but may occur as a result of faulty feeding.

Symptoms

Progressive swelling of facial bones occurs (*see* plate 4.7), the bones are soft and 'rubbery'. It has been seen in goats fed on high cereal diets with little green food.

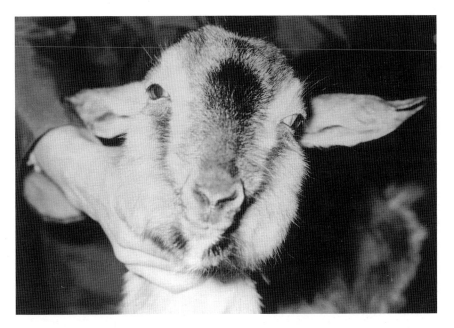

PLATE 4.7   Osteodystrophia fibrosa, showing the swollen cheeks

Treatment
Correct the diet to restore the normal ratio of 2:1 calcium to phosphorus.

DEGENERATIVE JOINT DISEASE

In cattle, especially housed bulls, a form of arthritis occurs as a result of the excessive feeding of calcium. It is also described in goats, especially bucks, which are never subjected to the heavy calcium losses of pregnancy and lactation. The symptoms are stiffness and a reluctance to move, becoming progressively more severe with age. To avoid the problem care should be taken not to over-feed calcium to housed bucks. Dairy rations are of course formulated for lactating animals and adult males do not require such large quantities of calcium.

BENT LEGS IN GOATS

In Australia a condition described as 'bent leg' developed in young pedigree bucklings aged four months. The forelegs bent inwards or outwards but the animals were in good condition. Experiments suggested that a calcium/phosphorus imbalance was the cause.

IRON

It is extremely unlikely that goats would ever be deficient in iron unless as a complication of the effects of blood-sucking worms. Trials have been carried out on kids to investigate a possible response to extra iron but it was shown to be of no benefit.

Chapter 5

PROBLEMS ASSOCIATED WITH GRAZING

INTERNAL PARASITES

ROUNDWORMS (PARASITIC GASTROENTERITIS)

Roundworms that infest the stomach and intestines can be a serious problem in goats. They probably represent the biggest challenge to the goatkeeper of grazed animals (to distinguish them from keepers of intensive goats that remain indoors all the time).

In nature, being a browsing animal, the goat would rarely be troubled by gastro-intestinal worms. Many methods of keeping goats compel them to graze and it is therefore not surprising that these worms have such a harmful effect.

They cause damage by sucking blood (e.g. *Haemonchus contortus*) or by reducing the absorption of digested food materials from the gut (e.g. *Trichostrongylus spp*). Reduced appetite has also been shown to result when they are present in large numbers. The deleterious effects, of course, lead to reduced milk yield and smaller weight gain. Inapparent or sub-clinical infestations are thought to be common, which means that the goat does not perform quite as well as she would have done without the worm burden.

The Physical Appearance of Roundworms
There are various families of worms that infest goats, including strongyles, trichostrongyles and nematodirus. They vary in length from 5 to 30 mm, some being visible to the naked eye.

The Epidemiology (or Pattern) of Disease
Despite the fact that there are many different species of gut

103

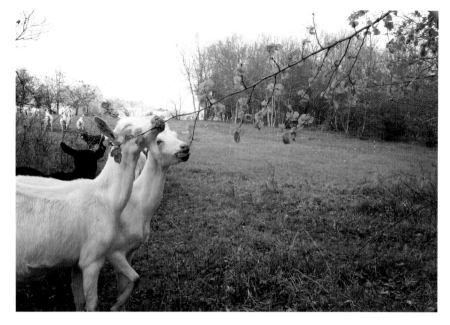

PLATE 5.1   Because of its height there is little chance of browse being contaminated by worm larvae

roundworm, we can put them into two types as regards the pattern of disease they produce; firstly the Strongyloides and secondly Nematodirus.

The Challenge to Goats
Goats acquire the infective larvae of these roundworms from the herbage of the pasture as they graze (*see* Figure 5.1). The larvae pass into the stomach or intestines and remain there, quickly maturing into adult worms. The adult worms then feed (causing damage to the gut) and eventually reproduce and lay eggs. The eggs pass out in the droppings of the goat on to the pasture. The eggs hatch and produce larvae which eventually become infective to other goats.

Disease caused by worms only results when the animal takes in large numbers of infective larvae at one time. A 'trickle' of infection does no harm; in fact it is probably beneficial to the goat, because it stimulates immunity.

Temperature and humidity influence the development of larvae on the pasture: hot, dry weather kills larvae; warm, moist

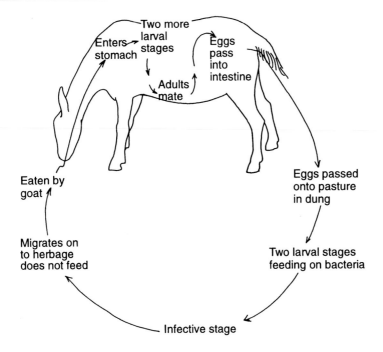

FIGURE 5.1   *Life cycle of the gut roundworm in the goat*

conditions help their survival. This means that the weather dictates when the larvae are ready to infest goats. Weather conditions are general for the region and therefore influence the development of all larvae. If the conditions are just right, all the larvae are infective at the same time and impose a sudden, heavy challenge on the grazing goat. Because weather conditions from year to year follow a similar pattern we can predict, fairly confidently, when pastures are dangerous. Thus we can list certain danger periods and suggest ways of avoiding disease. There are more than one 'group' of larvae each year, and consequently there are several danger periods. Three separate groups of larvae present a different source of challenge.

The Sources of Challenge

- Roundworm larvae which have overwintered resulting in a generation of infective larvae on the pasture in late winter.
- The increased numbers of infective larvae resulting from more eggs being poured out by does after kidding. This results in a

peak of challenge mid July.* This post-parturient rise is a phenomenon seen in goats and sheep when their output of parasite eggs increases dramatically. Various mechanisms account for its occurrence: the parasites lay more eggs and the goat appears to become less resistant to infestation at this time.

- Larvae passed out over the summer resulting in a challenge in early September.

It is natural for grazing goats to have parasites and it is impossible to think of keeping them free from them. The aim of the goatkeeper is to 'live with' the worms but to avoid dangerous challenges.

Goats should be removed from dangerous pasture at these times indicated above and put onto clean pasture. See suggested worm control strategies later in this section.

NEMATODIRIASIS

The nematodirus worm is present in a small percentage of goats in Europe. This worm parasite behaves slightly differently from the Strongyloides, infestation passing from the kids of one year to the kids of the following year. Thus, if the pasture is used for young kids every year, problems may arise. In fact, in Europe most kids are reared indoors and only go out to pasture when the threat of disease has disappeared. Goatkeepers in either of the following categories may have kids at risk.

- Those who graze kids from birth on the same pasture every year.
- Those who kid very early in the year and turn kids out to the same pasture in April or May each year.

In these instances, if nematodirus is known to be a problem, pasture management should be directed at providing clean pasture in the 'danger' period. Another alternative would be to house the kids and feed forage such as hay. The danger periods are illustrated in Figure 5.2.

---

* N.B. The above is typical for the UK. In warmer climates the challenge would be earlier, perhaps late May.

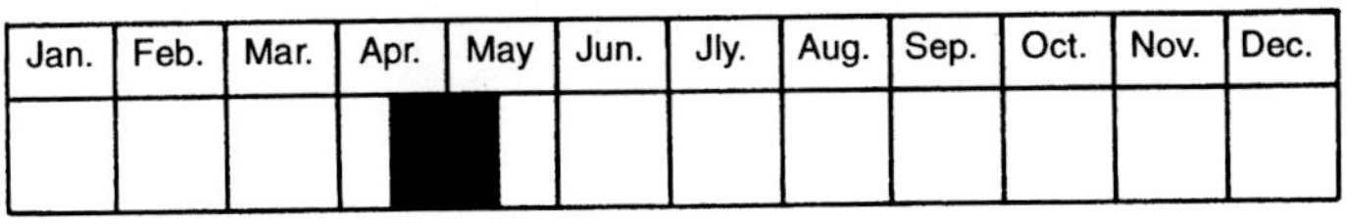

Jan.	Feb.	Mar.	Apr.	May	Jun.	Jly.	Aug.	Sep.	Oct.	Nov.	Dec.
			█								

FIGURE 5.2   The danger period for nematodirus infestation

Symptoms

Symptoms of worm parasites may be either very mild or very severe. The type of symptom may also vary with the age of the goat, adults tending to be more resistant than kids. Symptoms may also depend upon the type of worm involved: stomach worms such as Haemonchus are blood suckers and they tend to cause anaemia. Intestinal worms such as Trichostrongylus cause irritation and hence symptoms of diarrhoea. Normally many species of worm are present at the same time and so a mixture of symptoms are noticed. Goats suffering from a light challenge may show a loss of body weight or, in young kids, simply no increase in weight. More obvious changes may be noticed with larger numbers of worms, including 'staring' coats (dry, with the hairs standing up as if cold), reduced appetite and perhaps diarrhoea. Lactating does may have milk yields below their expected performance. Goats with very severe worm problems are generally in poor bodily condition, weak, anaemic[*] and have diarrhoea. In cases of acute (i.e. sudden) heavy challenge, animals previously in good condition may show rapid decline and become weak over a matter of days. Diarrhoea would probably be a marked feature.

Worm counts

Sometimes counts of the worm population of the goat are made at post mortem examination. This can be extremely useful if large numbers of goats are involved. As it enables the goatkeeper to take targeted action on the rest of the herd.

Treatment

Tremendous strides have been made in recent years in the field of anthelmintics. Modern preparations are safe and extremely

---

[*] The colour of the mucous membrane of the eye will give one an indication of severe anaemia (see plate 5.2).

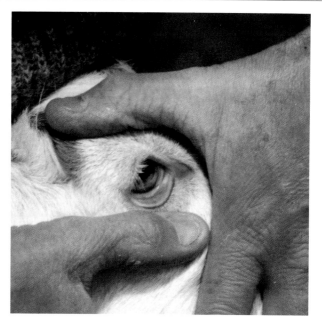

PLATE 5.2   Examination of the mucous membrane
of the eye – normal animal

effective. Even goats suffering from very severe disease can be cured by dosing with these drugs.

Basic Principles for the Control of Gut Roundworms

- Where roundworm parasites are concerned, sheep and goats are affected by the same ones and thus they should be considered together.
- All species of worm behave in the same way and thus can be considered as one type for practical purposes (except for nematodirus).
- Control is aimed at providing the goats with a clean pasture and if possible removing them from dangerous pasture.
- Drugs given to goats to rid them of parasites (anthelmintics) should be avoided as much as possible and kept in reserve. The worms are becoming resistant to them and it is unlikely that

new anthelmintics will be developed to replace them. Worm control relying on anthelmintics is not sustainable in the long term (*see* page 112).

- Plough and re-seed after each grazing year. This is obviously expensive and only suits certain farms.
- Grazing alternate species and cutting for hay or silage.

The roundworm parasites of cattle and horses are not infectious to goats. If possible this fact should be exploited to help control the roundworm parasites of these species. For example, grazing a pasture with goats, removing them to a clean pasture such as a hay aftermath and then grazing the goat pasture with horses will help to 'clean' that pasture. The horses can eat the infectious larvae that would be a threat to the goats, with no ill effects. Similarly, goats following horses grazing will not be harmed by parasites deleterious to the horses. The same is true of cattle in relation to goat parasites. One would have to consider the Johne's disease status, however, (*see* page 133) because this bacterium is a disease common to cattle, sheep and goats. (Sheep and goats must not be considered alternative species in this respect because they share the same parasites.)

Pasture that has been grazed by goats then allowed to grow for hay or silage could be considered 'clean'. By removing the

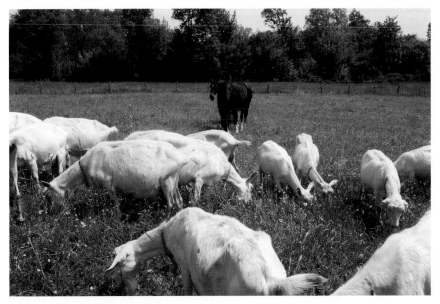

PLATE 5.3   Horses grazing pasture after the goats have grazed

herbage the pasture is cleaned and the drying action of hay-making means that the hay will also be 'clean'.

Try to avoid the goats grazing the pasture for longer than three weeks (by back-fencing if necessary). This will prevent the goats taking in dangerous levels of larvae produced from the worms that they were carrying. This number of weeks will be longer in cooler times of the year because the development of the larvae is temperature-dependant.

These suggestions will never entirely remove the threat of internal parasites but they are a logical step towards reducing the challenge and hence the requirement for anthelmintics.

Just as with vegetable gardening a rotation can be devised, for example:

Goats graze	Horses graze	Hay/silage	Goats graze	Horses graze	Hay/silage

FIGURE 5.3

Or, if no alternative species is available.

Graze	Hay/silage	Graze	Hay/silage	Graze	Hay/silage

FIGURE 5.4

The second rotation will depend upon the climate and its suitability for frequent hay/silage crops.

Goatkeepers with just one paddock might consider dividing it in order to cut one third for hay whilst the other two thirds are being grazed or left to grow for hay (*see* below).

Graze	Grow	Hay
Grow	Hay	Graze
Hay	Graze	Grow

FIGURE 5.5

This may help to avoid the main danger periods.

There are many variations and possibilities, for example, woodlands, cereal fields, aftermaths and post-harvest vegetable fields can provide a 'clean' break for the goats, in order to avoid 'danger' periods.

Suggested Worm Control Strategies

The Commercial Herd on a Large Acreage
In the ideal situation where pastures can be alternated each year with cattle or horses or an arable crop

- Continue to graze them as long as the weather allows.
- Take regular samples for faecal egg counts (FEC) (*see* page 116).
- Be prepared to dose in September if necessary.

In the commercial herd where no resting of pasture is possible
Pasture has been grazed by goats in the previous autumn and hay or silage aftermaths are available.

- Turn out in the spring.
- Graze goats until the end of May or June.
- Move in June when an aftermath becomes available.
- Keep moving to clean aftermaths from hay or silage.
- Continue to monitor faecal egg counts until housing.
- Dose only if recommended by your vet after examining the FEC result.

The Small Herd Grazed Continuously on One Paddock

- Dose after kidding.
- Monitor Faecal egg counts. Dose if necessary.

The Verge-grazed Goat
Ensure that the goat is moved continuously and avoid grazing the same area for twelve months. After a year's rest the ground will be free from parasites. No dosing is necessary in this situation.

The Stall-fed Goat
The goat is probably free from parasites but equally she is all the more susceptible, because she has poor immunity. Parasite control will depend upon what is fed and where the forage comes from. The following points may be of value:

- Browse can be considered to be free from parasites.
- Hay can be considered to be virtually free from parasites.
- Grass cut and fed from grassland where goat-house manure is spread *may* be dangerous but not likely. The danger can be reduced by composting the manure before spreading.

ANTHELMINTICS

These drugs are 'anti-helminths', active against helminth (parasitic) worms. The effect they have on the worms is to kill them either by starvation, or by causing paralysis of the worm in the gut. There are many compounds available and your veterinary surgeon will give you guidance as to which one to use. The modern drugs are extremely effective at getting rid of the worms from the goat's stomach and intestines. Some of them have the added bonus of controlling lungworms and liver fluke.

Anthelmintic resistance (AR)
With the increasing problem of anthelmintic resistance, veterinarians and farmers must completely re-consider how and when these drugs are to be used. The stark reality is that it is unlikely that any new compounds will be produced to replace the anthelmintics that we have at present. The way we have used them in the past is not sustainable and we must now be aware of the following. You would be advised to discuss this matter with your veterinarian and devise an action plan for your farm.

1. To avoid introducing resistant populations of worms with brought-in animals, quarantine the newcomers off pasture (for a few days). You may wish to discuss dosing them with your vet.
2. Adult grazing goats are generally immune to worms and only need worming in exceptional conditions.
3. Always check the weight of the heaviest animal and dose the whole group at that weight (because under-dosing speeds up resistance to anthelmintics).
4. It is possible (and a good idea) to check for AR in your goats by taking pre and post-treatment dung samples.
5. If you know the internal parasites on your farm you can use less drugs by targeting the problem accurately.
6. Discontinue the old rule of 'dose and move to clean pasture' as this will increase the development of AR. Delay the move for a few days after the dosing. Discuss this with your vet.

The Anthelmintics
There are three groups of broad spectrum wormers:

1. Benzimidazole (BZ) or 'white' drenches.

Anthelmintics Used For Goats

| Drug | Trade names | Activity spectrum | | | | Caprine dose‡ | Withholding time | |
		Gut round-worms	Tape-worms	Lung-worms	Fluke (adult only)		Milk days	Meat days
Fenbendazole	Panacur	*	*	*		10 mg/kg	7	28
Oxfendazole	Systamex	*	*	*	*	10 mg/kg	—†	28
Albendazole	Valbazen	*	*	*	*	7.6 mg/kg	—†	28
Ivermectin (oral)	Oramec	*	*	*	*	*	—†	28
Levamisole	Various	*		*		12 mg/kg oral	—†	28

Benzimidazoles

*Indicates the drug is active against parasite.

†Do not use in lactation.

Although all these drugs are widely used in goats, none of them are licensed for use on goats in the UK. Each country has different rules and regulations. Goatkeepers must check the manufacturer's directions and/or contact their vet.

‡Dose recommended by French researches.

2. Levamisole/Morantel (LM) 'yellow' drenches.
3. Macrocylic Lactones (ML) 'clear' drenches.

The anthelmintics within the groups are similar so if resistance occurs to one it is best to use an anthelmintic from another group. Your vet will guide you on this selection. When using the white or clear drenches, withhold food for up to 12 hours before drenching, if possible. This allows the maximum effect of the wormer.

Giving Anthelmintics

Administration can be either by injection, drenching or in-feed. For commercial herds a dosing set is used (*see* below) but for individual goats a large plastic syringe can be conveniently used (without the needle of course). (See plate 5.5.)

The injectable wormers carry some risk and are possibly best avoided. Goats are fussy eaters and in-feed preparations are very

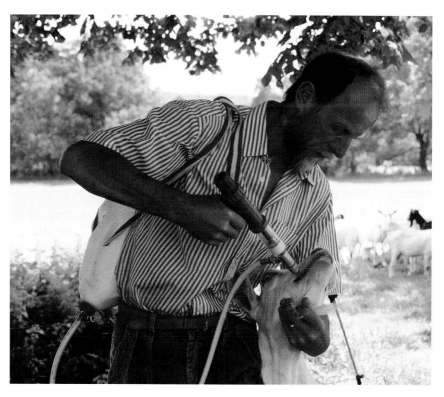

PLATE 5.4   Worming – using the oral dosing gun

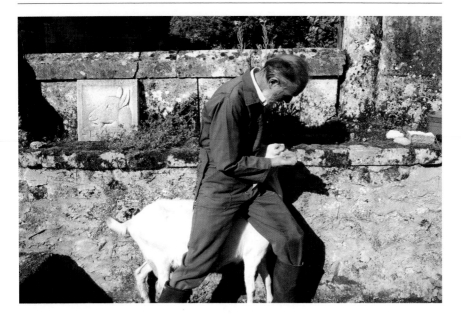

PLATE 5.5   Orally dosing the goat using a syringe

variable as to how much each goat consumes. Read the manufacturer's instructions carefully because some drugs have a milk-withholding time when milk should not be used for human consumption.

Dose rates
French researchers point out that goats metabolise away the drugs more quickly than sheep. Thus a higher dose rate should be applied to goats than that stated on the manufacturers information. They recommend double the dose given to sheep for the white drenches. For ivermectin, they suggest an increase of 50 per cent above the sheep dose rate.

SOME OTHER POINTS ABOUT WORM CONTROL

Paddock rotation
Some years ago scientists attempted to combine efficient grazing management and worm control. The concept of a series of six paddocks was proposed which the sheep (or goats) grazed in

rotation, spending about one week in each paddock. After six weeks they returned to the first paddock and repeated the cycle. Although sensible from a grassland management point of view, it can be disastrous as a method of parasite control.

Stocking Rate

Once a certain minimum number of animals is reached for an area of grassland, parasites become a potential danger. Thought must be given to parasite control and it makes little difference whether twenty or thirty goats are grazed there because the number of infective larvae that can result from just one goat grazing a paddock is very high. It is the timing of exposure to the parasite that is important. If the goats are all moved from the pasture at the right time, then no serious challenge or disease results.

Worm-free Goats

Outside the laboratory, it is neither practical nor desirable to have 'worm-free' goats. A healthy goat is one that experiences a small amount of challenge but avoids the danger periods when the pasture is heavily contaminated with larvae.

The Effects of Worming Goats

The administration of anthelmintics (white and yellow drenches) to goats removes the population of worms established in the goat at that time. If the goat is then returned to infected pasture she immediately starts to take in infective larvae. Thus another population of adult worms is established within her, in the space of about 4–6 weeks. With the clear drenches there is a longer persistence of the drug but eventually re-infestation occurs.

The lifespan of a worm.
Based on studies in sheep, the average life is thought to be about 3 months. After this time they die naturally.

Worm Egg Count (Faecal Egg Count – FEC)

Parasitologists have attempted to quantify the severity of parasite infestation by counting the parasite eggs present in a gram of faeces. Results expressed in the form of say '500 eggs per gram' are thought to indicate more serious infestation than one of '100 eggs per gram'. Faecal egg counts can be used to estimate the worm burden of a group of goats. Your vet will help you with the interpretation of them. It must be stressed that these counts are a useful piece of extra information but only as a guide and they must be interpreted with care. Most studies into them have been based upon sheep flocks. Low FECs can be sometimes misleading.

How to collect samples for FECs
In a large herd, grouping the goats on a clean area of concrete or pasture and holding them there for 10 minutes will suffice. After that time, using polythene bags, collect a few pellets from six or eight different piles of fresh pellets. Send them to the lab in the individual bags.

Worm egg counts are useful to determine whether there is a problem of anthelmintic resistance. A faecal sample is taken before and after dosing with the wormer. If the anthelmintic is working, the result should be almost negative by 48 hours after treatment. In this procedure it is important to mark the goats that have been sampled and sample from the same goats individually for the second test.

Infestation in Indoor Reared Kids
Kids are extremely susceptible to worms, and on account of their habit of soiling feed containers it is possible to spread larvae via contaminated feed. Always ensure that feed and water containers are kid-proof and cannot be contaminated.

LUNGWORM

The symptoms of lungworm disease are coughing goats which, in severe cases, fail to thrive. The worms inhabit the air passages and cause inflammation (parasitic pneumonia). Two species of worm can be responsible for these symptoms, *Dictyocaulus filaria* and *Muellerius capillaris*. Both worms are present in the United Kingdom, the United States and France. *M. capillaris* is much more widespread than *D. filaria*.

Dictyocaulus filaria
This worm can infest both sheep and goats, but there is generally little disease associated with it in goats. It has a similar life cycle to the gut roundworms, except that the adults inhabit the lungs, not the intestines. Thus there is an extra stage of migration by the larvae from the intestines to the lungs, via the bloodstream. The life cycle of this worm is illustrated in Figure 5.6.

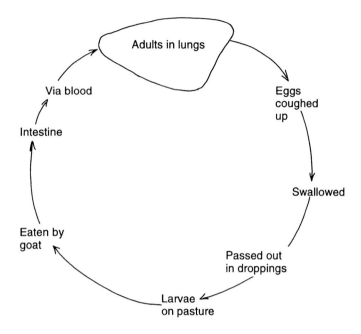

FIGURE 5.6   The life cycle of the lungworm, D filaria

Muellerius capillaris

Although this is a parasite of sheep and goats, it rarely causes disease in sheep but can cause disease in goats. In Britain many goats are thought to be infested by this parasite, but this does not necessarily mean that they are suffering disease. Disease symptoms include coughing and increased breathing rate. The life cycle of this worm is complex and includes an intermediate host such as a snail or a slug. It is generally found on wet pastures.

The Patterns of Lungworm Disease

Disease associated with both worms can be considered together. Coughing is generally seen in late summer or autumn. Because the parasites are picked up while the goats are grazing, disease is generally seen at pasture. It may also be encountered in stall-fed goats when forage is fed from fields previously spread with goat or sheep manure.

In a report from New Zealand, a large study revealed over a third of goats' lungs were affected by lungworm. By comparing affected and non-affected carcase weights, researchers found a difference of between 0.75 kg and 1.5 kg between the two groups. This suggests that the lungworm was responsible for some reduction in growth rate.

Control
The principles of control are similar to those for gut roundworm. Challenge arises mainly from the pasture in early summer, resulting from both overwintered larvae and larvae from infested adults. (In the case of *M. capillaris* it is from larvae harbouring in the snail or slug.) Therefore goats moved and dosed as suggested for gut worm control should avoid lungworm disease. Development of immunity against lungworm infestation is much better than it is against gut roundworms. This probably accounts for the relatively low prevalence of disease. Most goat owners can afford to be relatively unconcerned about lungworm disease in goats for the following reasons:

- Infestation with *D. filaria* is relatively rare, and it generally causes little disease.
- Grazing control measures applied for gut roundworms should also control lungworms.
- Some anthelmintics used to control gut roundworms are also effective against lungworms; they include albendazole, oxfendazole and ivermectin.

LIVER FLUKE DISEASE (FASCIOLIASIS)

The fluke is a parasite of the livers of ruminants such as the goat and sheep. Adult flukes inhabit the bile ducts of the liver and they can remain there for months or years. In the case of *F. hepatica* an intermediate host, the mud snail (*Limnaea truncatula*), is necessary for the completion of the life cycle of the fluke. The snail only lives in wet, poorly drained areas and so liver fluke disease tends to be prevalent in the high-rainfall regions of the world and in irrigated pastures. Both *Fasciola hepatica* and *Dicrocoelium dendriticum* can infest goats. In Turkey, goats are sometimes found carrying both species at the same time.

The Life Cycle
A diagrammatic illustration of the life cycle of the liver fluke is shown in Figure 5.7.

The adult fluke is a hermaphrodite possessing both male and female organs. It lays eggs which pass into the bile and out with the goat's droppings. Hatching of the eggs occurs if the temperature is above 10°C and miracidia are released. The miracidia swim about in search of a snail and if they are successful they penetrate the tissues of the snail.

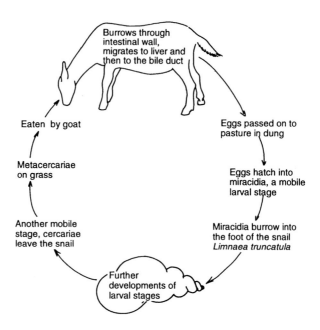

Burrows through intestinal wall, migrates to liver and then to the bile duct

Eaten by goat

Metacercariae on grass

Another mobile stage, cercariae leave the snail

Further developments of larval stages

Eggs passed on to pasture in dung

Eggs hatch into miracidia, a mobile larval stage

Miracidia burrow into the foot of the snail *Limnaea truncatula*

FIGURE 5.7   The life cycle of the liver fluke, Fasciola hepatica

Several stages of development take place within the snail and after a minimum period of about five weeks cercariae are released on to the pasture. The cercariae swim in the moisture on the pasture finally settling on blades of grass. They then become covered by a secretion which hardens and they remain on the grass as metacercariae. The metacercariae are ingested, along with the herbage, as the goat grazes.

The Pattern of Fluke Disease
Weather conditions have a profound influence upon the disease and the amount of disease varies from year to year. The amount

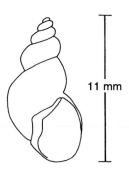

FIGURE 5.8   Shell of the Limnaea truncatula

11 mm

of challenge to the goat is dependent upon the survival of the mud snail. Thus the factors that influence the survival of the snail determine the disease threat. The two key factors are temperature and rainfall. A temperature of 10°C is essential for the development of the snail, and adequate rainfall is necessary. These two criteria are generally present in the summer in the wetter parts of Britain but to varying extents. It is possible, however, to measure these two parameters over the early summer months and then produce a forecast of the severity of the challenge that can be expected that autumn and winter. Goat-keepers can use the forecast to avoid disease in their goats.

The Use of the Fluke Forecast
If the year has been wet, then the time that the goats are liable to take in parasites is from late August through to December. Thus, all pastures can be safely grazed from spring until the middle of August, irrespective of how many snails are present. If the fluke forecast is 'bad' the goats should be moved to well-drained pasture which is unlikely to have any fluke present. On the other hand a 'good' fluke forecast means that there is going to be little challenge that year and such precautions need not be taken.

Jan.	Feb.	Mar.	Apr.	May	Jun.	Jly.	Aug.	Sep.	Oct.	Nov.	Dec.

FIGURE 5.9   The danger periods on pasture where fluke is a problem (in a 'bad year')

Control

In theory fluke can be controlled by three main methods:

1. Eliminating the snail is achieved by either drainage, or the use of molluscicides such as copper sulphate. Both methods are expensive and have to be carried out thoroughly. The use of molluscicides also has an environmental contamination risk. For the majority of goatkeepers with only a few animals they are not worthwhile from an economic point of view.
2. Preventing the goat ingesting the parasite by avoiding grazing in dangerous times and planning grazing accordingly. It is difficult for goatkeepers who have no alternative grazing to use. The stall feeding of goats on hay, greengrocers' trimmings or other forage may be an answer in bad years.
3. Eliminating the fluke in the goat's liver can be achieved through the use of drugs active against fluke in the live animal (flukicides). These not only remove the parasite from the liver but also reduce the number of fluke eggs that are deposited on to the pasture. This in turn reduces the challenge to goats in subsequent grazing years. It would seem sensible for goat-keepers who graze fluke-infested pastures to use Albendazole as their standard anthelmintic. This wormer has the added bonus of removing adult flukes from the liver. This advice would be modified if anthelmintic resistance were present on the farm.

Symptoms

Liver fluke disease can manifest itself in either of two forms: acute or chronic.

Acute fluke disease

Eating massive numbers of the parasite over a short time results in large numbers of immature flukes passing from the gut of the goat into the liver. Acute disease results from the damage caused by the tremendous sudden injury to the liver. The symptoms are sudden and death can occur in a very short time. In less severe cases the goats are dull, off their food and may kick at their abdomens in pain. If post-mortem examination is carried out, the liver is seen to be enlarged, bloody and friable.

Chronic fluke disease

More common than the acute form, chronic disease is seen in the late winter. Affected animals become progressively weak and lose weight. Diagnosis is confirmed by the demonstration of fluke eggs in the droppings of the goat.

Treatment
Various drugs are available to treat this disease, though none of them are licensed for use in goats. Nitroxynil (Trodax) is an injectable preparation. Albendazole (Valbazen) is an anthelmintic which is also effective against fluke although only in the adult form. However, it can be used in goats.

Black Disease (Infectious Necrotic Hepatitis)

Black disease has been recorded in goats. The disease causes sudden death in adult goats. It results from an infection with *Clostridium welchii* in conjunction with fluke migration through the liver. Routine vaccination of goats should avoid this problem.

Tapeworms

Many species of tapeworm can inhabit the small intestine of goats. They include *Moniezia expansa* which is found throughout the world. This particular species has a mite as its intermediate host, the goat becoming infected by eating mites while grazing.

The Significance of Tapeworm Infestation
To my knowledge little research work has been carried out to investigate the harmful effects of tapeworm infestation in the goat. On the surface, one would assume that harm may be caused but there is little evidence to support this hypothesis in sheep, where the problem has been studied. My opinion is that tapeworm infestation in adult goats is of little or no significance but may occasionally be important in kids.

Diagnosis and treatment
Diagnosis of the disease is made by examination of the goat's droppings. In the unlikely event of problems an anthelmintic such as albendazole (Valbazen) can be used for the treatment of affected kids.

OTHER DISEASES AND EXTERNAL PARASITES

GRASS TETANY (HYPOMAGNESAEMIA/GRASS STAGGERS)

See Chapter 6, 'Problems Associated with Milking Goats', page 143.

FOOTROT

This is a specific lameness of grazing goats and sheep, commonly seen in the summer months and occasionally during the winter, in housed animals. Typically infection enters the hoof at the skin horn junction (*see* Figure 3.3) and causes inflammation of the sensitive laminae. The infection spreads below the hoof causing severe pain and lameness. Because it affects both sheep and goats it is relevant to point out the widespread distribution of this disease in sheep flocks.

The Bacterium Involved and Predisposing Factors

All cases of footrot are associated with infection by *Bacteroides nodosus*. The predisposing factors to the infection are damp, lush pasture, typical of that found in the United Kingdom and many temperate regions of the world. The moisture of the pasture has a tremendous bearing on the distribution of the disease. It is noticeably absent from the arid regions of the world. The effect of the moisture is to soften the hoof horn, allowing the bacterium to penetrate more easily. *B. nodosus* can persist in the hooves of infected animals for years, but in the pasture it can only live for about a week. This is very important if you are trying to avoid the problem, and I shall discuss this under 'Control'.

Symptoms
Lameness is slight at first and there is only a small amount of swelling between the claws. As the horn is underrun and the sensitive laminae become involved lameness becomes increasingly severe. Typically there is a foul smell associated with it and the horn begins to separate from the underlying tissue. The animals are reluctant to walk and may graze on their knees. Milk yield may fall and some animals will lose weight.

Treatment

Apply antiseptic agents in order to remove any infection. These are best applied topically on to the affected area. This is achieved, in a small number of goats, by using formalin or zinc sulphate in a plastic container and dipping individual feet. In a large herd a foot bath could be employed.

In severe cases your veterinary surgeon may prescribe anti-bacterial drugs, by injection. Avoid paring the feet at this stage but do it a week after the bathing.

Requirements for the Treatment of Footrot

- Hoof shears
- A race and footbath (for a large herd)
- Local antiseptic, either 3% formalin or 10% zinc sulphate solution
- A hard surface such as concrete or stones.

After bathing the feet the goats should be left to stand on a hard, dry surface for as long as possible (minimum of thirty minutes), in order to allow the antiseptic to work. You should not immediately turn them out into a muddy field. When the job is completed clean the equipment in 5 per cent formalin (or its equivalent) and collect the hoof trimmings. If any of a herd are affected then the whole herd should be put through a footbath (*see* page 64). As goatkeepers are well aware, goats dislike water and forcing them through a footbath is not an easy job. Foot bathing should not be carried out more than once a week because it is detrimental to horn and skin.

Persistently affected goats may be best culled because they act as a reservoir of infection for the pasture and hence the rest of the herd.

Control

1. *Attempting eradication by pasture management* Because *F. nodosus* only survives for a maximum of ten days on pasture it is possible to eliminate the infection from fields. This can be achieved by carrying out the treatment as detailed above, on say three occasions, with an interval of ten days between each. The goats must not be returned to the same pasture until ten days have elapsed.
2. *Vaccination* There is a commercial vaccine called Footvax (Schering-Plough) available for sheep, which can be used in

goats. No work has been carried out to test its effectiveness in the control of footrot in goats, but I feel that it is worthwhile using in problem areas. The primary course of immunisation comprises two injections separated by an interval of six weeks. The manufacturers recommend this should be started in October. Single booster injections should be given twice-yearly in October and February each subsequent year.

PINK EYE (CONTAGIOUS OPHTHALMIA, NEW FOREST EYE)

As the name suggests, this problem is an eye infection that spreads in herds of goats (and sheep). The conjunctiva or membrane that covers the eye becomes inflamed. In severe cases the cornea, lying below the conjunctiva, is involved. This is a disease of the summer when the agents that spread the germ abound. It can be spread by flies, dust and long grass. At colder times of the year, feed troughs are probably responsible because they cause crowding of the goats, allowing direct contact between them.

Symptoms
At first a watery eye is noticed with excess tears spilling over on to the skin. There may be some reddening and the cornea becomes cloudy. Over the course of a few days the discharge thickens and becomes sticky. Recovery generally occurs within a fortnight, but very occasionally, ulceration of the eyeball may occur, with loss of its fluid.

Treatment
Some cases will recover without any treatment but your veterinary surgeon may supply you with an antibiotic ointment to aid healing and reduce the risk of spread to other goats. Application of the ointment should be made several times a day but check the directions supplied.

Control
The organism generally associated with this condition is *Rickettsia conjunctivae*. Abroad, *Neisseria ovis* has been recorded as contributing to the condition. Recent work in the United States has revealed that a mycoplasm, called *Mycoplasma conjunctivae*, may also be involved. These agents are present in the eyes of some goats. They act as reservoirs of infection for other goats when conditions are right for spread. Thus the only control

measures that can be applied are to treat affected animals quickly, isolate them and avoid crowding goats when the disease is present in the herd.

FLUORIDE POISONING (FLUOROSIS)

Grazing pastures contaminated by fluoride can cause poisoning in goats. In the United Kingdom this is most common in pastures near brickworks. The fumes from the brick making process deposit fluoride on to the pasture. Certain parts of Bedfordshire are renowned for this contamination. The symptoms include lameness and stained teeth. There is no treatment, and in such situations goatkeepers would be advised to run a 'flying herd', that is, to buy in milkers each year. This avoids rearing replacements which become diseased at a young age.

FLY STRIKE (MIASIS) AND MAGGOT INFESTATION

Any open wound in the summer months attracts flies. Certain flies, the blowflies, actively seek such wounds in which to lay their eggs.

After hatching, the larvae of the blowfly eat the tissues of the unfortunate goat, causing intense irritation and discomfort.

Treatment
Larvae should be removed and the wound cleaned. A dressing incorporating an antiseptic preparation should then be applied. The wound should be examined twice a day until healing has occurred. Ivermectin preparations by injection may be useful.

Control
Examine and dress all skin wounds, being careful to inspect for signs of fly eggs, or larvae. Remove all predisposing causes of wounds such as projecting nails. Treat diarrhoea promptly in the summer months because this attracts the flies.

The use of insecticides to prevent fly strike
In my experience goats rarely require such measures but spraying them with a compound used for sheep would be effective. There are no UK licensed products for goats but 6 per cent cyromazine is used for prevention of fly strike in sheep. It could

be applied to goats but not in females producing milk for human consumption. Pour-on preparations are available, discuss this with your vet.

WARBLE FLIES (HYPODERMATOSIS)

Warble flies can affect goats overseas: *H. lineatum* was found in goats in Turkey, but this species is not now present in Britain. The condition is characterised by the appearance of swellings under the skin of the back. The swellings on the back are the developing larvae. When developed they fall to the ground, pupate and the adult fly then emerges. Veterinary advice should be sought before treatment.

THE NASAL FLY (*Oestrus ovis*)

The larvae of this fly spend part of their development in the nasal cavities and sinuses of sheep and goats. The sheep is the specific host but occasionally goats may be affected. In the United Kingdom the fly is only active in the summer months and it is not generally a widespread problem. In hotter parts of the world, the fly is active for longer periods and one South African survey revealed that three-quarters of goat herds were infested. The adult flies can cause distress to the goats by pestering them.

Life cycle
The adult fly deposits its larvae around the nose of the goat and the larvae migrate into the nasal cavities. After several weeks they pass into the sinuses and when the goat sneezes they fall to the ground. After pupating on the ground the adults mate and commence to deposit larvae. The cycle is then repeated.

Symptoms
The adult flies upset the goats when they are grazing. The larvae irritate the linings of the nose causing the goats to sneeze and produce a discharge. In my experience the effects on the goats are fairly minimal.

Treatment
Various organophosphorus compounds are reported to be effective. Ivermectin (Ivomec) (Merial) has recently been used to treat

it in sheep and is effective in goats at a dose rate of 0.2 mg/kg by injection. Other members of the Macrocylic Lactones (ML group of wormers) are also used in sheep for treatment of this parasite.

TICKS AND TICK-BORNE DISEASE

Ticks are large parasites that feed periodically on sheep and goats, dropping off from the animal when they have taken a meal of blood. Depending upon the species of tick involved, another stage may subsequently attach and feed the following year. Although unsightly, their main damage is to spread disease when they bite the goat (*see* LOUPING ILL, page 130). In problem areas such as the south-west of the United Kingdom, routine dipping or spraying of goats may be advisable. Alternatively, the odd tick can be treated individually by applying insecticide locally. It is best not to pull off the tick because the mouth parts often remain in the skin, although special 'hook' removers can be successfully employed. Even in the warmer areas of Europe, the tick does not seem to affect the goat very much.

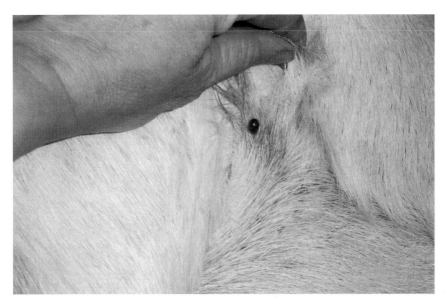

PLATE 5.6   Tick on a goat in spring

LOUPING ILL (ENCEPHALITIS)

Louping ill is a viral disease that causes an inflammation of the brain of sheep. It is transmitted by the bite of a tick infected with the virus. Very occasionally it may cause disease in goats, though there are no reports of clinical cases. A survey carried out on feral goats in Scotland revealed that many of the goats had antibody to the disease which suggests that it probably occurs from time to time.

The symptoms in sheep are those of fever, convulsions and paralysis. It is only likely to occur in hill areas where ticks abound. Control depends upon control of the ticks.

ORF (CONTAGIOUS PUSTULAR DERMATITIS, CONTAGIOUS ECTHYMA)

This is a highly infectious viral disease of goats and sheep. It causes scabby sores around the lips and muzzle. The disease can pass from sheep to goats and vice versa. Although rapid spreading, it is generally not a serious disease except that it does result in loss of productivity. Whereas in sheep flocks it predominantly affects young lambs, in goats it seems to cause problems in all ages of stock. It is a common disease throughout the world.

Symptoms
Initially, swellings and pustules occur which soon become scabby and crusty. They are especially common at the corners of the mouth. Most cases are fairly mild; the scabs become dry and fall off, so that the wound is healed over in about three weeks.

Loss of condition occurs because the goats are disinclined to eat on account of the pain. The yield of milking does may fall. Grazing animals tend to suffer more than goats fed quantities of concentrate food. Kids can be quite seriously affected, especially if bottle fed.

Transmission
Spread occurs by direct contact with other animals or through inanimate objects such as fences and feeding troughs, which have been contaminated by infected animals.

Treatment

It is doubtful whether treatment helps at all but the application of creams and ointments may reduce the spread of orf around the herd. Offering some concentrate food will help to avoid any setback in grazing goats.

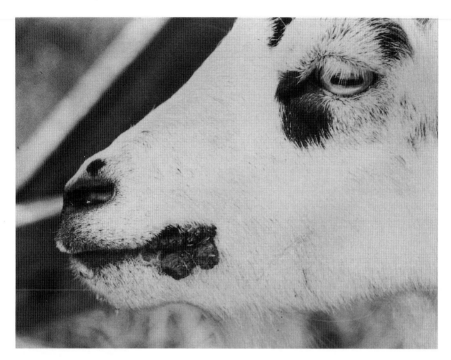

PLATE 5.7   Symptoms of orf on a goat's mouth

Control

Isolation of affected goats may reduce the spread of the disease. Vaccination may be of value in the early stages of an outbreak. Scabivax orf vaccine (Schering-Plough) is only licensed for sheep but can be used in goats. The vaccine generally comes in 50 dose packs and is only economic for goatkeepers with several animals. The vaccine is given by scratching the skin with a special applicator dipped in vaccine. Do the vaccination either inside the thigh or preferably under the tail.

When to vaccinate

- Does 8 weeks before kidding
- Kids from vaccinated dams, at 15 days
- Kids from non vaccinated dams, at birth.

The virus can persist for many years in the scab and therefore outbreaks may occur after several years of freedom from disease. It is unnecessary (and not desirable) to use the vaccine unless problems have occurred with this disease in former years. In Zimbabwe orf appears to be more severe in goats affected by concurrent caseous lymphadenitis.

Human infection
Humans can become infected and painful sores develop in the

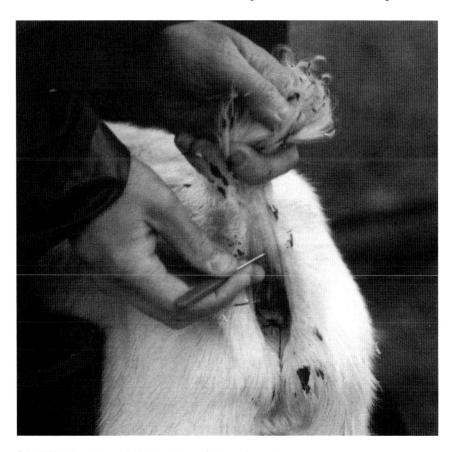

PLATE 5.8   The administration of the orf vaccine

skin. Care should be taken when handling affected animals or when administering the vaccine.

GID, STAGGERS (COENURUS CEREBRALIS INFESTATION)

If the larval stage of the dog tapeworm, *Taenia (Multiceps) multiceps*, develops in the goat's brain, this disease may result. As the cyst grows it causes pressure and damage to the brain cells of the goat.

Symptoms
The symptoms seen depend on the part of the brain involved. Affected goats may circle, show a high-stepping gait, or blindness in one eye. If the cyst lies in the spinal cord, posterior paralysis may result. Occasionally, a softening of the skull may be noticed where the cyst lies beneath the bone. It may be necessary to use X-rays to confirm that the cysts are present in the skull.

The cycle of infection
Infected dogs put out tapeworm eggs in their faeces. Goats grazing contaminated herbage eat the eggs and the larvae migrate to the brain. Dogs become infected by eating uncooked carcasses which contain tapeworm cysts.

Control
Cook sheep and goat offal before feeding it to dogs in order to destroy the tapeworm cysts and administer tapeworm treatment tablets to dogs that come in contact with goats and sheep. Your vet will guide you on the selection of a dog wormer.

Treatment
Treatment of the goat will rarely be possible and slaughter will probably be necessary.

JOHNE'S DISEASE (PARATUBERCULOSIS)

Johne's disease is a chronic incurable infection of the intestines of goats, sheep and cattle. It is caused by *Mycobacterium avium* subspecies *paratuberculosis*, or *Map*. It is a slow-growing bacterium belonging to the same family as tuberculosis. Infection causes a thickening of the intestine with the consequence that less nutrients are absorbed. Johne's disease is a worldwide problem. In Norway 9 per cent of goats were found to be infected in a post-mortem survey. The UK prevalence is not known but it is fairly frequently diagnosed in submissions to the Veterinary Laboratories Agency.

Possible link with human disease

It has been suggested that the organism may also be a possible cause of Crohn's disease in Humans. Such a causal link has yet to be proved or disproved.

Symptoms

Loss of flesh is the main symptom, the goat gradually becoming emaciated. The droppings may become slightly loose but diarrhoea is rare. It may be that cases of 'the fading goat syndrome' are due to Johne's disease. Loss of appetite and milk yield are reported but often the appetite remains good. The weight loss, despite good nutrition, is quite striking and the goats tend to develop a poor dry coat.

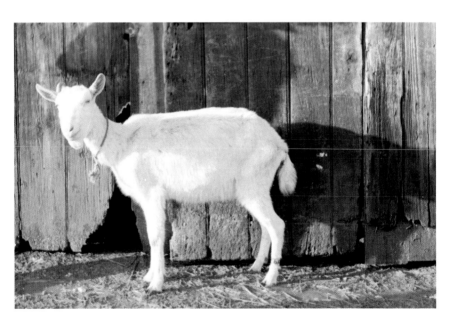

PLATE 5.9   Johne's disease

Treatment
There is no treatment for Johne's disease; affected animals should be slaughtered as soon as possible after they are diagnosed. This helps to prevent the spread to other animals.

Diagnosis
The initial diagnosis is made using a direct smear from the faeces and microscopic examination. At post-mortem examination, enlarged mesenteric lymph nodes are found with characteristic caseous lesions. (*See* below.)

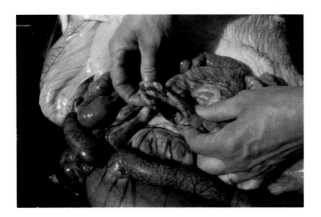

PLATE 5.10   Johne's disease – post mortem, showing incised, swollen, mesenteric lymph node. The node contains a small quantity of (white) caseous material. The findings were confirmed by laboratory examination of the lymph node

Control
New experiences of the control of Johne's Disease, emphasise the need to take action on many fronts at the same time. The important factors to remember about the disease are:

- The organism can survive on pasture for up to a year.
- Infected animals may put out bacteria on to the pasture in their droppings, for months before the symptoms are noted.
- Tests for Johne's disease are unreliable in picking out the infected animals, before they contaminate the premises. The culture of faeces, however, does speed up the process of identifying infected animals. Tests on the blood are useful but not one hundred per cent reliable.

- Being a chronic disease (incubation period of up to 4 years), the wasting symptoms are not usually manifest until the animal is an adult, by which time, it may have infected several others.
- Control on the infected farm is very difficult. Sometimes the slaughter of a herd must be considered. Even if one does get rid of the herd, the farm cannot be restocked with ruminants for at least a year, otherwise the new animals may become infected.

Positive actions to be taken in an infected herd

- Vaccination is effective, but must be carried out early on in the the life of the young kid (i.e. under one month). Your veterinary surgeon will order it for you. Plan ahead, to make sure it is in stock in time for your new kids.
- Cull animals with symptoms as early as possible, in order to reduce the contamination of pasture.
- Use faecal culture in an attempt to search out the infected animals.
- In order to avoid maternal transmission to the kid, 'snatch rearing' should be practised. The kid is removed from the mother immediately after birth to prevent faecal contamination from a possibly infected mother. The colostrum is then taken from the mother and offered to the kid, after warming to body temperature. Take at least a litre off the goat, and feed it to the kid over the first 24 hours. On day two, start to mix the mother's colostrum with a powdered milk replacer, and over two days get the kid on to the milk replacer. This will reduce the risk of maternal transmission to the offspring, which is the most important route of infection. The kids are then best reared away from adults for as long as possible, before they join the herd.
- Avoid pooling colostrums from several goats.
- The manure from affected animals' quarters would be best spread on arable land, and not on grazing land. Manure should at least be composted to reduce risk of pasture contamination. The best method is to stack the manure and allow it to heat up. After some weeks turn it and then stack it again. Do not graze pasture for 3 months after spreading infected manure.
- Grazing horses (which are not susceptible to Johne's disease) after goats may help to reduce re-infection to subsequent goats grazing the pasture.

Buying-in stock

Because Johne's disease is so difficult to eradicate from a premises, all goatkeepers should try to avoid purchasing infected stock. It is always worth enquiring from the vendor of a goat whether or not he or she has had any animals with the condition. It is also important to remember that infected cattle, sheep or deer can infect goats. You may consider screening new purchases for Johne's disease. When new goats are purchased, isolate them, take 10 g of faeces from each to your vet to send off for a faecal culture test for Johne's disease. Faecal culture is more efficient than direct smears but not foolproof because the germ may only appear in the faeces intermittently. Alternatively, blood samples may be tested.

Note for Veterinarians

The agar gel immuno diffusion test (AGIDT) is thought to be as accurate as faecal culture in detecting infected animals. A 7 ml blood sample from each goat should be submitted along with faeces.

PHOTOSENSITIVITY

In certain circumstances goats exposed to several hours of sunlight may develop changes in the skin, which can vary from slight thickening to very severe damage. Photosensitisation occurs only when certain photodynamic substances are present in the skin. In the presence of sunlight an allergic type of reaction occurs, resulting in a thickened skin and dermatitis. This condition only occurs if the goats are white or have white patches of skin, the explanation for this being that they are unpigmented. Photosensitisation should not be confused with sunburn which usually appears some time after exposure to sun.

Substances predisposing to photosensitisation

Many plants that goats eat have a propensity to cause this disease directly, for example, St John's wort (*Hypericum perforatum*). Other plants can cause problems indirectly, if the liver is damaged or not working efficiently. The breakdown products from these plants (phylloerythrins) accumulate in the tissues of the body, including the skin, instead of being excreted. Such plants include the lupin (*Lupinus angustifolius*); other plants giving similar problems include kale (*Brassica rapa*) and lucerne (*Medicago sativa*).

Symptoms
Thickening occurs on the white (unpigmented) parts of the coat especially around the ears and muzzle. White goats, such as the Saanen are particularly prone to this condition. The skin thickening is especially noticeable on the backs of the goats and to a lesser extent on the sides. In very severe cases the skin is shed. The affected goats may show signs of irritability and excitement.

Treatment
Once removed from the direct rays of the sun the goats soon recover. Putting them in a shed for a week or two should be all that is required in mild cases. If the skin is very badly damaged then your vet may prescribe drugs to reduce the inflammation and control any infection that may develop. By removing the goats from the pasture and putting them inside, one normally prevents the goats having access to the plants involved.

PINE (COBALT DEFICIENCY)

Pine is a wasting disease caused by deficiency of cobalt in the feed (*see* COBALT DEFICIENCY, page 97). Cobalt is essential in very small quantities and hence its designation as a trace element. The condition is found mainly in areas of the world deficient in cobalt. Pine is relatively uncommon in British goats; I have rarely seen it, but other authors have described it. The low prevalence of pine is accounted for by the facts that firstly, only certain soils are low in cobalt and secondly, the majority of British goats receive adequate attention and mineral supplementation. An important point in the pattern of the disease is the fact that cobalt cannot be stored by the goat and must be continuously available in small quantities.

Symptoms
Cobalt is essential for the production of vitamin B_{12} in the rumen. The vitamin B_{12} requirements of ruminants such as goats are quite high. Deficiency causes an inability to metabolise propionic acid and a failure of appetite. This loss of appetite results in loss of weight and eventually death.

Treatment
Affected animals respond well to the administration of either

cobalt or vitamin B_{12}. Cobalt sulphate is generally given, the usual amount being 10 mg by mouth, at weekly intervals. For convenience cobalt 'bullets' can be administered to adult goats. These lodge in the reticulum and slowly release cobalt to the goat. Because the reticulum is underdeveloped in young animals the bullets are not satisfactory for kids.

BLOAT (RUMINAL TYMPANY)

All goats above weaning age possess a large fermentation chamber called the rumen (*see* Chapter 4, page 75). Carbon dioxide and methane gases continuously produced from the fermentation are eliminated by the animal belching. If for some reason the gases cannot be got rid of, pressure builds up in the rumen. The left-hand flank of the goat becomes distended due to the enlarged rumen and the animal has great difficulty breathing. It is fairly uncommon in goats compared with cattle and sheep.

Bloat can result from many causes including:

- An obstruction of the oesophagus (*see* CHOKE, page 78).
- Paralysis (as in TETANUS).
- Eating foods which produce lots of gas, over a short period of time.
- Stable froth formation, associated with certain forages such as lucerne. In this condition the gas in the rumen remains as thousands of bubbles (froth) as opposed to one large collection of gas, and the goat is unable to belch these bubbles up. This is by far the most common type of bloat.

The reason why the gas bubbles tend to foam or froth is very uncertain. Many theories have been put forward and many explanations may be partially correct. The high surface tension of the bubbles can be partially explained by the composition of the food material eaten. For example, lush pasture with a high protein content has been cited. The quantity of saliva produced may also be important, because the saliva aids the breakdown of the froth. Occasionally, bloat develops in goats suddenly fed large quantities of concentrates.

Symptoms
Affected goats have distended left flanks. They may show signs of discomfort; kicking, bawling or grinding their teeth. In more

serious forms, the goats have obvious difficulties in breathing, because the abdominal contents restrict the space into which the lungs expand.

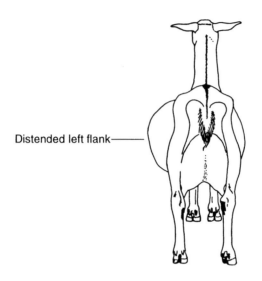

Distended left flank——————

FIGURE 5.10   *The effect of bloat on a goat's appearance*

Treatment
Preventing the animal eating anything is the first step to take. The type of treatment then depends upon the seriousness of the condition. If you suspect or can see a blockage in the oesophagus, call your vet and do nothing further, unless the goat is in great distress. If the animal is near to death then try puncturing the rumen with a stabbing action, using a sharp pointed knife (*see* plate 9.5). In very mild forms, relief can be given by drenching (carefully!) with 25 ml of vegetable oil such as peanut oil. 10 ml of washing up liquid could also be used in an emergency. Proprietary silicone-based drenches are also available. Alternatively your vet may pass a stomach tube in an attempt to release the gas. In acute cases more drastic action is required and the rumen may have to be punctured with a knife or preferably a trocar and cannula. This is inserted by a stabbing action with the trocar inside the tube of the cannula. Once in place the trocar is withdrawn to allow the gas out (see also pages 141 and 260).

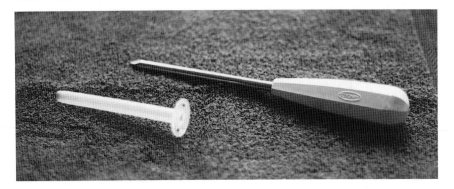

PLATE 5.11 The trocar and cannula

After-care
Because the treatment can interfere with the delicate rumen functioning, 'seeding' the stomach with live yoghurt may be beneficial. Feeding branches from fruit trees such as apple may help to improve rumen movement.

Prevention of bloat
Take care when grazing goats on rapidly growing pasture. Restrict the time of grazing to short periods, especially if lucerne is grazed. The goats may be drenched with vegetable oil before they are turned out on to pasture. Never turn hungry animals out on to rich pasture; fill them with hay before they graze for the first time in the spring.

HEAT STRESS

Heat stress can result when goats are exposed to strong sunshine in the summer months. It is especially likely to occur in tethered goats that are unable to seek shade. The symptoms are panting, rapid breathing and thirst.

Treatment
Move the goat into the shade as quickly as possible and offer it cold water to drink. If necessary, dowse the back of the animal with cold water.

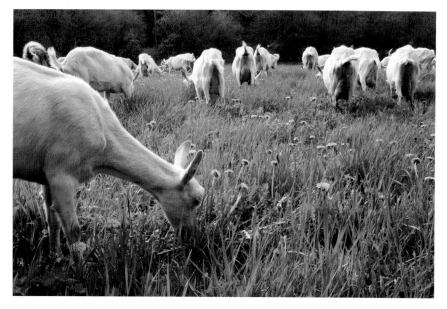

PLATE 5.12 Bloat prevention – take care when turning out in the spring

FOREIGN BODIES IN THE RUMEN (FOREIGN BODY PICA SYNDROME)

Sometimes goats ingest pieces of metal, nails, etc. when grazing. Reports from developing countries describe significant numbers being diagnosed. The objects, being heavy, tend to remain in the rumen and reticulum. Often sharp objects penetrate the wall of the rumen and cause damage and infection elsewhere. Symptoms are varied and include loss of appetite, depression, fall in milk yield and loss of weight. The condition is unlikely to occur in well fed animals but more in conditions of near starvation caused by drought, etc.

Chapter 6

PROBLEMS ASSOCIATED WITH MILKING GOATS

Two groups of problems are commonly encountered in goats producing milk:

1. Metabolic disorders
2. Diseases of the udder and teats.

They conveniently form a natural division in this chapter.

METABOLIC DISORDERS

Metabolic disorders result from a disturbed input-output balance of nutrients. At the start of lactation, milk production represents a sudden drain on the goat's reserves. Constituents such as protein, fluids and salts, are all lost from the body and the goat's metabolism has to cope with those sudden changes. Years of selection for high-yielding goats has resulted in animals capable of giving far more milk than is required by twins or even triplets. Thus the strain on the goat is made worse and it is hardly surprising that sometimes things go wrong.

MILK FEVER (HYPOCALCAEMIA)

This problem occurs in milking does at or around kidding, but it is fairly uncommon. A survey in 1964 revealed only five cases out of nearly a thousand animals. In the GVS survey (*see* page 276) only two cases were recorded. Milk fever is most likely to be seen in the age range of 4–6 years. In a study of forty goats with hypocalcaemia in Norway the time of onset was:

17% less than one week before kidding
25% during kidding and next few days
20% less than three weeks after kidding
37.5% more than three weeks after kidding.

The problem is essentially a disturbance of calcium metabolism. Calcium is abundant in the bones and teeth, with smaller quantities present in the blood and other tissues. The mineral is vital for muscle contraction, and if blood levels fall this function of enabling muscles to move, ceases.

The Biochemistry of Calcium

A basic understanding of the turnover of this mineral will help the reader to understand why milk fever occurs. Figure 6.1 is a diagrammatic representation of the movement of calcium within the lactating doe.

In the non-lactating doe some of the calcium present in the diet is absorbed into the blood and transferred to the bones for storage. Vitamin D influences this movement, together with the hormone calcitonin. When required, calcium can be released from the bones back into the blood under the influence of

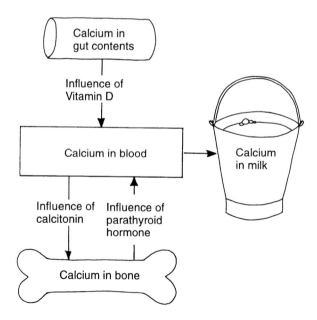

FIGURE 6.1   The movement of calcium in the lactating doe

parathyroid hormone. Problems arise in does around kidding, when the demand for calcium suddenly increases. Milk is high in calcium and therefore calcium has to be brought back out of the bones into the blood. It takes a little while for the gut to increase its absorption of calcium, even though there is adequate calcium in the diet.

Why Milk Fever Occurs

Hypocalcaemia simply means 'low blood calcium'. This does not mean that the goat is deficient in calcium, the bones are full of it. It simply means that temporarily the blood calcium level has fallen because the complex control mechanism described in Figure 6.1 has failed. At kidding the goat is suddenly called upon to produce in excess of 2–3 litres of milk each day. Milk is high in calcium and this obviously represents a heavy loss, which temporarily lowers the blood calcium level to less than half its normal value (from 2.48 to 0.94 millimole/litre).

Symptoms
Because calcium is essential for muscle tone, goats affected with milk fever appear to be weak. They generally lie down and become unable to rise. Cudding ceases and they do not usually pass water or faeces. If left untreated, the goat would probably become gradually weaker and eventually slip into a coma and die.

Milder forms may be quite common, being responsible for protracted kiddings. Symptoms of slight weakness (ataxia) affecting the gait, may also be noticed in about half of the cases. The temperature of the affected goat is frequently below normal (38°C).

Treatment
Response to the administration of calcium salts is good, the symptoms normally disappearing within a few hours. Calcium borogluconate is the commonly used injection which can be given either under the skin or directly into a vein. In acute cases, the best treatment is probably to give 25 ml of the 40 per cent solution into the vein and also inject a further 75 ml under the skin. This technique combines a rapid response with a deposit of calcium which can be slowly absorbed from under the skin.

After the injection of calcium borogluconate, the goat's body normally adjusts and mobilises its own calcium from the bones. If the doe is lying on her side, then she should be propped up with a bale so that she is lying on her breastbone (brisket). This prevents rumen fluid entering the lungs and prevents bloat developing. For the following two milkings it is best not to take off too much milk (as this will impose more strain on her).

Prevention of milk fever
Understanding the biochemistry of calcium enables us to realise what goes wrong and to rectify any faults. If calcium is fed in high quantities just prior to kidding, the control mechanisms register this high input. They send adequate quantities into the bone but also reduce the absorption of calcium salts from the intestine. If this mechanism persists after kidding, the calcium lost in the milk depletes the reserves, resulting in a state of low blood calcium. Conversely, if a diet high in phosphorus and low in calcium is fed for the week prior to kidding, the goat's metabolism is ready to adjust to the sudden change. In this situation, calcium is already being mobilised from the bones and milk fever does not occur. It is not easy, of course, to formulate the ideal low-calcium diet unless one consults a book on nutrition chemistry. Some values that may be useful, however, are the following:

	Ratio	
	(g/kg dry matter)	
	Calcium	*Phosphorus*
Hay (medium quality)	5.5	3
Lucerne	13	2.5
Sugar beet pulp	13	1

As a rule of thumb only investigate this further if cases of milk fever are occurring in your herd. Farmers whose cows have a known susceptibility to milk fever use vitamin D just before calving or even dose the cow with calcium gel at calving. There are no reports of their use in goats but they could be used in problem herds.

KETOSIS (ACETONAEMIA)

This condition can occur within the first month of lactation. It is very similar to pregnancy toxaemia (*see* page 84) and only occurs in housed, lactating animals, in the winter. Ketosis is basically the inability of the milking doe to keep up her potential for milk production, due to faulty management. Dairy goats have been bred for very high milk yields, this inherited attribute being termed 'genetic potential'. The doe can only yield that quantity of milk if her nutrition and management are just right. If the doe yields to her potential on an unsatisfactory diet, then something has to give and in this case ketosis develops. Ketosis results from any one of a variety of management errors, or a combination of them (*see* ACETONAEMIA, page 87).

HYPOMAGNESAEMIA (GRASS TETANY OR GRASS STAGGERS)

The word hypomagnesaemia means the condition of low blood magnesium. In normal animals a certain concentration of magnesium salts is present in the blood. When these are not present, symptoms of 'staggers' may be seen. It is mainly a problem of adult milking goats; it is not common.

Symptoms
The onset of symptoms can be very rapid. The goat behaves strangely, becomes unco-ordinated and 'staggers'. On closer examination the muscles can be seen to be contracted and the animal is excitable.

The predisposing factors
Ruminants are unable to store magnesium for long periods and the disease is an input-output problem. This is best explained by referring to Figure 6.2.

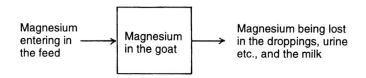

FIGURE 6.2 *Input and output of magnesium in the lactating doe*

The goat attempts to keep the magnesium in the blood constant but this is affected by variations either in intake of the food or in the output, for instance in the milk. Many factors can influence intake of magnesium in the diet, the obvious one being a change of diet. Three situations generally predispose to hypomagnesaemia; they are as follows:

- Lactating does grazing rapidly growing spring grass
- Heavy lactation
- Stress from poor weather (for example, no shelter in the winter).

Treatment
The administration of magnesium salts can completely reverse the course of this disease. They must be given in time, however, as the disease can be rapidly fatal. Magnesium sulphate is normally given under the skin, but occasionally your vet may administer some into the vein. Response to treatment can be fairly rapid, the goat being back to normal the following day. The injection of magnesium sulphate can precipitate a lowered blood calcium. It is therefore prudent to inject calcium borogluconate at the same time as the magnesium sulphate.

Prevention
As the disease occurs mainly in lactating animals, prevention is generally easy because they are handled twice a day. Ensuring that magnesium is present in their concentrate rations is the simplest method. If extra is required, calcined magnesite can be fed at 6g a day. Other methods available are the provision of licks or even giving the goats a 'bullet' which remains in the stomach. The bullet is impregnated with magnesium and if given by mouth, settles in the reticulum, where it gradually releases magnesium. Methods of administering magnesium in the drinking water are available for cattle. They could possibly be adapted for goats in very large herds.

DISEASES OF THE UDDER AND TEATS

Any impairment of function of the udder of the dairy goat is very serious. It is also not surprising that such diseases are fairly common, if one considers the following three points:

- Dairy goats have been selected for milk yield over the centuries and a goat with a large exposed udder has been produced.
- They are subjected to twice-daily milking which imposes a strain on the defence system of the teats.
- Goats are frequently milked one after another so that the possibility of transmission of germs from one udder to the next is very high.

Mastitis

Mastitis is an inflammation of the udder, almost always associated with germs and showing a great range of variation from mild to very severe. In the dairy cow, where the disease has been studied extensively, it has been demonstrated that inapparent or sub-clinical mastitis is very common. This can also be shown to occur in the goat. Thus, mastitis may be affecting the glands of goats when the owner does not even realise it! Mastitis is economically important because it reduces milk yield and it may also cause permanent damage to the udder.

Recognition of Mastitis – the Symptoms
1. *Sub-clinical* No visible changes in the milk or udder. Simple tests can demonstrate changes in the milk. Experiments have revealed a lowering of yield by affected halves.
2. *Mild* Clots in the milk.
3. *Acute* Swollen, painful udder. Clots and watery milk, reduced yield. The goat may be off her food. There may be blood in the milk. It is generally seen close to kidding.

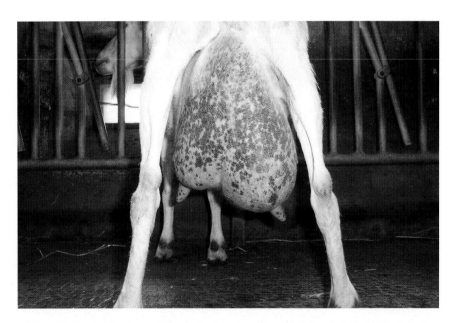

PLATE 6.1   Clinical mastitis, note the small size of the left (affected) half. This goat suffered permanent loss of milk from this half.

4. *Very acute*   The changes as in number 3; almost invariably blood is present, the udder may even feel cold and clammy. The goat is not eating and is a very sick animal, possibly too weak to rise. Her temperature is high. Gangrene of the udder may be the final outcome. It is generally seen close to kidding.
5. *Chronic*   Repeated episodes of number 2.

It should be noted that these observations are for guidance only and, of course, the goat may start with a mild mastitis which may progress to the acute form.

How Common is Mastitis?
There are few figures available for the prevalence of mastitis in goats. One survey revealed that in large herds 25 per cent of goats can have one infected half. One Indian report recorded 32 cases out of a flock of 140 goats. In an investigation in Greece, nearly half the udders were found to be infected. A chronically infected herd in Norway contained 28 goats with mastitis out of 50. Many of these cases were, of course, inapparent or sub-clinical mastitis. In a small survey carried out by the author, only five cases of clinical mastitis were recorded in 231 adult goats over a year (not all of them were lactating). A 1964 United Kingdom survey revealed that clinical mastitis was responsible for large losses.

In summary, I conclude that sub-clinical mastitis is common and perhaps more common than is realised.

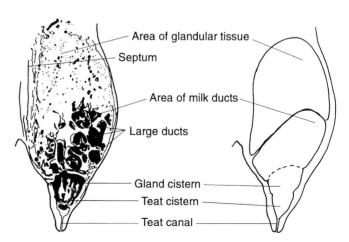

FIGURE 6.3   Anatomy of the udder and teats (vertical section of one half)

Figure 6.3 illustrates the basic anatomy of the udder. The two halves are separated by a septum of fibrous tissue, which means that infection from one side does not spread to the other side.

The Spread of Mastitis

Micro-organisms, especially bacteria, are always present in an attack of mastitis. They almost always enter by way of the teat canal, ascend the teat duct and invade the glandular tissue. Because these bacteria are incapable of moving on their own accord something must allow them to gain entry to the teat. Thus, there are two important aspects of mastitis: the presence of bacteria and, more importantly, the factors which allow them to invade the teat. The two main sources of infection are:

- The environment of the goat (including the bedding and the contaminated external surface of the udder and teats).
- Other goats with mastitis.

Factors Predisposing to Mastitis

The factors which allow the bacteria to invade are thought to be many and varied and the situation is very complex. Below is a list of such factors, although many of them are disputed or not proven.

1 Physical injury
    - Bushes
    - Fences
    - Butting by other goats
2 The milking process
3 Overmilking
4 Machine milking
    - Incorrect vacuum pressure
    - Teat cup liners
    - Vacuum fluctuations
5 Housing and bedding
6 Teat sores

In summary, it is known that the above factors do influence cases of mastitis but scientists are frequently at a loss to explain how they have this effect.

The Effects of Mastitis on the Mammary Gland

Once the bacteria have invaded the gland they begin to multiply very rapidly, because they are in an ideal warm moist medium.

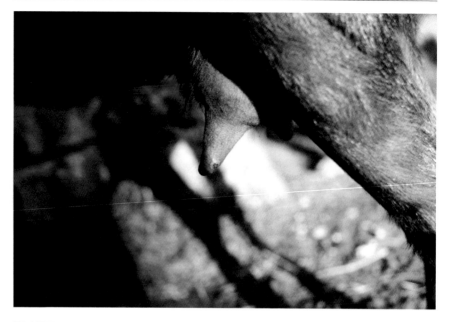

PLATE 6.2   Teat sore

The udder attempts to defend itself by producing defence cells which eat up (phagocytose) the bacteria. Frequently this defence system is enough to overcome the infection. Many such cases of sub-clinical mastitis are eliminated without the goatkeeper ever knowing that they occurred. If, on the other hand, the weight of infection is too great, the bacteria continue to multiply and their presence inflames the cells of the gland, destroying them or changing the nature of the milk they produce. In very acute cases the inflammation is so great that blood and pus appear in the milk. Goats with very acute mastitis develop a temperature as a result of the inflammatory process in the udder.

Diagnosis of Sub-clinical Mastitis and Cell Counts
Several indirect tests are available to help diagnose this problem. They are cheap, simple to use and results are available immediately. They are based upon chemicals which demonstrate the presence of white blood cells, the existence of which indicate that mastitis is affecting the udder.

By definition one cannot see sub-clinical mastitis, one can only demonstrate the changes in the milk by biochemical tests and bacteriology. In dairy cows one method of demonstrating the presence of sub-clinical mastitis is to count the number of 'cells' in the milk. These cells originate from the gland tissue itself and from the white blood cells which flood into the mammary tissue is response to infection of the gland. Thus in cows one can 'quantify' the level of sub-clinical infection by the 'cell count' i.e. a count of 50,000 cells per ml is more severe than a count of 30,000 cells/ml. This simple and useful relationship is now being applied to goats milk. Commercial goat dairies now use cell counts on the bulk milk to gauge the quality of the milk in a dairy herd. A good result would be in the band < 1,500,000 cells/ml and a poor result > 2 million. It can be seen that the range for cell counts in goats is much higher than for dairy cows.

The technique can also be applied to individual goats to identify chronically affected animals that are best treated or culled.

Infective Agents Associated with Mastitis
Many different types of bacteria can be isolated from cases of mastitis in goats. The following list stresses the fact that many organisms can be associated with caprine mastitis:

> *Streptococcus agalactiae, S. dysgalactiae, S. pyogenes, S. zooepidemicus, Staphylococcus aureus, Staph. epidermidis, Staph. pyogenes, Yersinia pseudo-tuberulosis, Enterobacter cloacae, Pseudomonas aeruginosa, Clostridium perfringens* type C, *Corynebacterium ovis, Bacillus cereus, Klebsiella pneumoniae, Mycoplasma putrifaciens*

In most outbreaks it is rather academic to know which type is involved for three reasons:

1. Treatment should be initiated early on, before laboratory test results are available.
2. We are aware that the types of bacteria in the goat's environment are legion and the circumstances which allow them to gain entry are more important than knowing which organism happened to invade the gland.
3. Broad spectrum antibiotics (or combinations) are used for treatment and the choice often depends upon the history of success on each enterprise.

Treatment
Mild, and even more acute cases, respond well to therapy with antibiotics, infused directly into the affected half. It must be

realised, however, that permanent damage in the form of destroyed gland tissue may have occurred. In such cases, the gland may well secrete less milk in subsequent lactations. Very acute cases may not respond well and the infection may even kill the goat. Sometimes the episode will be so severe as to make the doe useless as a producer of milk, even though she recovers.

Milking does

Infection during lactation is helped by the fact that the milk flushes out the organism but is hindered by the fact that the antibiotic used as treatment is also flushed out.

Dry does

The reverse applies for cases occurring in dry does where there is very little flushing effect.

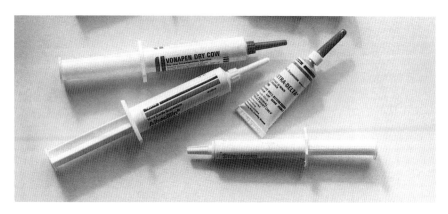

PLATE 6.3   Intramammary tubes and syringes

Preparations

All the preparations for the treatment of mastitis are supplied in intramammary tubes or syringes which are designed for use in the dairy cow but can be used in goats. There are a plethora of them available containing a wide range of different drugs.

In the absence of specific recommendations for goats it is probably best to use a cow dose, that is one tube for each half being treated. On no account give in to the temptation to economise by using half a tube for each half, as you may spread infection from one half to the other via the intramammary tube. Your veterinary surgeon will prescribe for you enough repeat infusions to establish a cure. The number of repeats is determined by the type of drug used and the base which it is in, being either quick or slow release. There is an obvious dilemma in treatment between obtaining a satisfactory cure and attempting to avoid the waste of milk. Milk must be discarded because it contains drugs. Observe the instructions given on the tube as to how long the milk must be discarded after the last treatment. Administration should be undertaken as hygienically as possible. The milk should be stripped out before doing so.

Clean the end of the teat with cotton wool soaked in alcohol (spirit) or antiseptic. Insert the nozzle into the teat, squeeze out the contents and then try to massage the ointment up the teat, sealing the end with the finger and thumb. In goats with tiny teat apertures it may be necessary for your vet to use a cat catheter in order to put the antibiotic into the teat.

Alternatively try infusing the tube contents without inserting the nozzle into the teat. Simply hold the nozzle in close

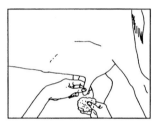

After milking, clean teat with cotton wool and spirit

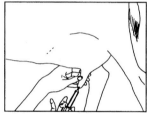

Insert the nozzle fully into the teat canal and apply steady pressure on plunger to deliver the full dose. Or use close apposition method

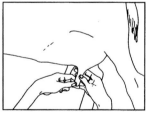

Hold the end of the teat and massage the teat, moving the antibiotic upwards into the gland

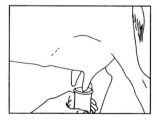

Immerse the teat in teat dip

FIGURE 6.4   Administration of an intramammary tube

apposition to the hole in the teat orifice, and squeeze the tube/plunger. The ointment will normally run into the teat without any problems. It may also help if the tube is warmed very slightly or taken from a warm room temperature before infusing.

Taking Samples for the Laboratory
Sometimes it is beneficial to take milk samples for examination at a laboratory. This is done in the case of a serious herd outbreak or in order to check the suitability of an antibiotic drug that has been prescribed (sample before it is administered). Cleanliness is essential if the sample is to be of any value, and the following steps should be observed. A badly taken sample may be contaminated and cause more confusion than no sample at all.

1. Obtain a sterile container from your vet or lab.
2. If teat is dry, remove dirt by wiping.
3. Discard the first stream of milk into another container.
4. Clean the end of the teat with cotton wool soaked in spirit (e.g. methylated spirit); wait for the spirit to dry.
5. Discard the next few streams of milk.
6. Collect the sample.
7. Label and date the sample, then send it to your veterinary surgeon/ laboratory.

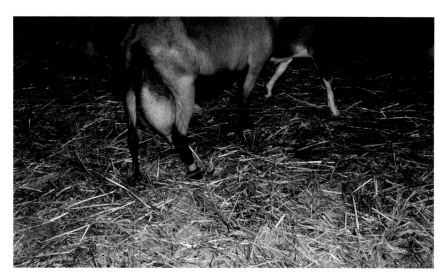

PLATE 6.4   Leg identification helps identify treated goats

Prevention of Mastitis

For as long as people milk goats, mastitis will always occur. Just treating the symptoms, that is clinical cases, will only solve part of the problem. It is necessary to avoid sub-clinical mastitis, which is very prevalent, but not noticed. This means preventing new infections.

As vaccines are of no use in this role, new infections must be prevented either by **better husbandry** or by **breeding**. Unfortunately, there is little prospect of dairy goats being selected for mastitis resistance. If this type of breeding is pursued, other, less favourable characteristics may be produced or good traits lost. It is also probably the case that the high-yielding, easy-milking goat, is the most prone to mastitis. She is also, of course, the goat most breeders are striving to produce. Perhaps in the long term there is a case for selecting goats with moderate yield, capable of producing from forage, instead of from the heavy concentrate diets that are used at present. Unfortunately the economic considerations of present day production don't favour low input, low output methods.

A. The Control of Mastitis by Better Husbandry Designed to Prevent New Infections

In the dairy cow, mastitis control by this approach has been very successful. The same principles apply to goats and I know goatkeepers who have achieved success by using better hygiene and husbandry. This can be achieved in many ways. On page 151 the predisposing factors to mastitis were listed. Each point will now be covered.

Physical injury to the teats
The dairy goat does not have a lot of ground clearance and thus attention must be paid to detail to avoid mechanical damage to the udder and teats. Door steps and bedding retaining boards can cause injury. Grazing scrub areas is potentially dangerous with 'low slung' goats. Play and aggressive behaviour may result in udder damage. Sometimes this can be avoided by keeping groups of goats separate.

The milking process
This should be carried out quietly, efficiently and hygienically.

The doe becomes conditioned to being milked and therefore helps in the process by 'letting down' her milk. In fact milk let-down is not a conscious act but is a reflex that follows stimulation of the teats and even the familiar stimuli of, for example, seeing the milker. The pathway of the reflex is partly transmitted by the nerves and partly by the action of the hormone oxytocin. The oxytocin acts by squeezing the alveoli which contain much of the milk and sending it down into the gland cistern. Myoepithelial cells actually contract and squeeze the alveolus.

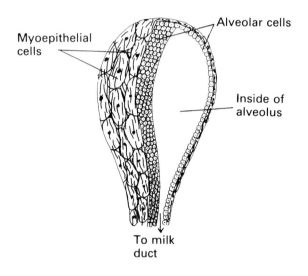

FIGURE 6.5   The alveolus and myoepithelial cells partly cut away

The importance of a regular routine at milking
The importance of all this to mastitis is that this milk let-down reflex is prevented by fear, excitement, stress or pain. For example, change of routine at milking or the presence of a noisy visitor tends to inhibit the reflex and thus prevent efficient emptying of the udder. This means that the doe has to be milked for a long period in order to obtain the milk and this causes damage to the teats.

Overmilking
It seems obvious that excessive milking of goats will result in damage to the teats. This has been a widely held theory in dairy

cows but not conclusively proven by experiment. Avoiding excessive stripping would seem a sensible precaution, however. If the goat is milked to excess, then very slight damage to the teat canal results, which predisposes to bacteria entering. Research has shown that infection mainly takes place immediately after the milking; thus any steps taken to reduce stress to the teats at this stage is beneficial.

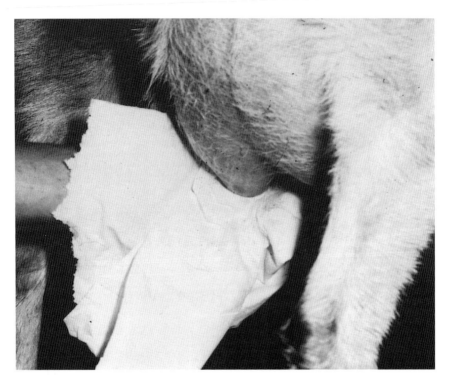

PLATE 6.5   Udder washing

Hygiene
The importance of being clean at milking cannot be over-emphasised for two reasons. Firstly, to avoid contamination of the teats and secondly to assist clean milk production. Remember that most infections occur immediately after milking and thus the cleaner the teats are, the smaller the chance of infection. Udder cloths should be disposable and not used for one goat after another. In the opinion of many, including the author, visibly

'clean' teats in goats, say, at pasture, need not be washed before milking.

The use of teat dips

Because most infections take place immediately after milking, the application of antiseptic to the teats just after milking has been shown to prevent new infections. The teats are immersed in teat dip as soon as they have been milked and this temporarily sterilises them. This gives the teat time to recover from the milking process and to regain its protective function.

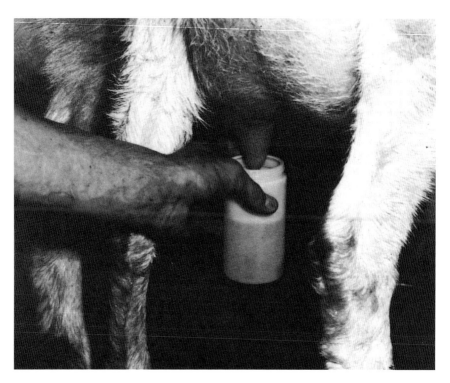

PLATE 6.6　Teat dipping

Machine milking

There are several aspects of this milking method which predispose to mastitis. Firstly, damage can occur to the teats as a result of using a machine. This can arise from faulty vacuum pressure, excessive vacuum fluctuation or worn teat cup liners. The machine should be checked regularly to ensure that these faults are corrected.

The second aspect about the machines is that they can physically carry infection from one doe to the next. Clinical cases of mastitis should always be milked last and the machine carefully sterilised afterwards.

Housing and bedding
Bacteria capable of causing mastitis are around the goat all the time. It is obvious that the cleaner we keep them, the fewer the bacteria that will be present on the teats. Of equal importance is the state of the bedding as regards physical damage to the udder and teats. Cold, wet concrete chills udders; clean straw bedding does no harm at all.

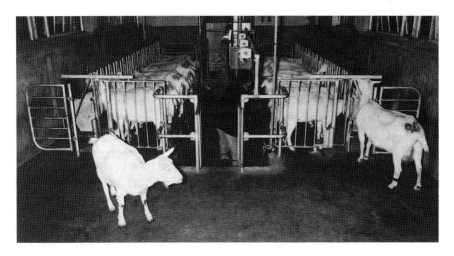

PLATE 6.7   The milking parlour at the former National Institute for Research into Dairying

Teat sores
Cuts, chaps and sores on the teats not only cause problems at milking because the goat is in pain but they also provide hiding places for bacteria. Care should be taken to avoid such sores and prompt treatment should be given in the form of udder creams. More serious, infected sores require the application of ointments containing an antibiotic. If large numbers of animals are affected, your veterinary surgeon should be consulted, in order to identify the cause and to suggest ways of control.

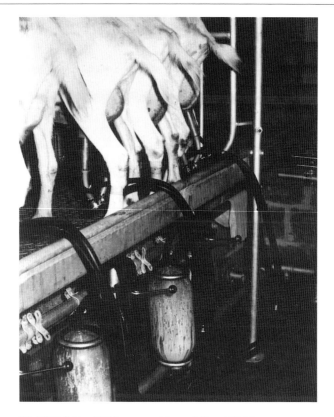

PLATE 6.8   Milking machine at the NIRD

B. Prompt Treatment of Existing Infections
By treating existing infections quickly, the goatkeeper reduces the reservoir of infection that poses a threat for the other goats in the herd.

Dry Doe Therapy
This practice is widespread in the dairy cow. At drying off all udders are infused with antibiotics which persist in the udder for several weeks. The rationale for its use in cows is that many infections carry on from one lactation to the next and cause severe disease just after calving. The dry period is a good time to eliminate the infection because no milk has to be thrown away and the antibiotic remains in the udder for a long period. This practice can be applied to goats in just the same manner. I have reservations about using antibiotics in this way because it is no

logical answer for the long term. In my view greater emphasis should be placed upon good husbandry and breeding for goats with sensible yields. These goats are less prone to mastitis. However, it may be prudent to use dry doe therapy in goats that had mastitis during the previous lactation.

The Sale of Goat's Milk

Goatkeepers do have the moral obligation to sell wholesome, fresh milk that is fit for human consumption. They must also make themselves aware of the laws concerning the sale of milk or milk products. Never sell milk from goats with mastitis because raw goat's milk is often fed directly to infants. Some bacteria associated with mastitis are a human health hazard if drunk. Milk containing antibiotic residues (from does being treated for mastitis) must never be sold. Some people are allergic to certain antibiotics and drinking contaminated milk can make them very ill. Antibiotics in milk may induce resistance in bacteria and thus reduce the effectiveness of antibiotics when given to humans for medical purposes. Always take careful note of the milk-withholding time given on the mastitis treatment, and take the advice of your prescribing vet.

Induction of Lactation

Lactations are reported to be induced by a 50 mg sub-cutaneous implant of Hexoestrol.

CUTS AND LACERATIONS OF TEATS

These can be very important and very frustrating problems to deal with. Very serious cases should be referred to your veterinary surgeon immediately. The most serious ones, frequently torn on barbed wire, are those that penetrate the teat canal. This can be easily seen if milk is leaking from the wound. Mastitis may develop if infection gets into the gland through the wound. From a practical point of view, milking a goat with a cut on its teat is difficult and time-consuming, for the obvious reason that the wound is painful. Unfortunately if the goat is to continue to produce milk then she must be milked. This action, of course, delays the healing of the wound. Very severe cuts will be stitched up by your vet but superficial ones may respond to the application of sticking plasters. Vets may use superglue to bring together the edges of some wounds. A serious teat wound should

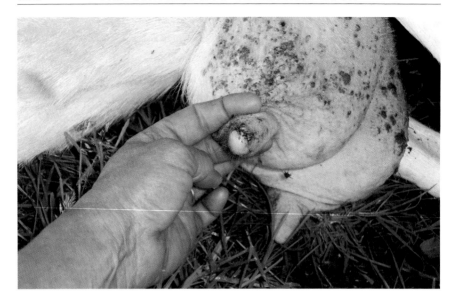

PLATE 6.9   Sutured teat – post dog attack

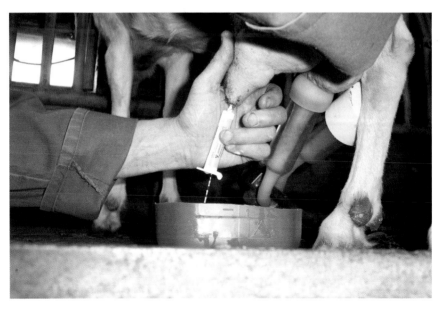

PLATE 6.10   Sutured teat – draining milk using sterile, empty I/M syringe
case

be considered very carefully. After treatment (sutures, plasters or just cleaning) it may be best to dry off the affected side in order to avoid a chronic open wound developing. If this course of action is followed, an antibiotic intramammary tube is inserted before drying off (discontinuing milking). The next lactation sees the affected side come back into milk. Your veterinary surgeon will almost always prescribe a course of antibiotics, if the wound includes the teat canal. This is to safeguard against mastitis developing.

Prevention
Avoid putting goats into areas that contain objects capable of damaging their udders. Clear up bits of barbed wire and check fences regularly to ensure they are goat-proof. Try to avoid situations where goats will be tempted to jump through barbed wire fences – for example, hungry goats or goats in season.

OEDEMA (DROPSY) OF THE UDDER

Some does develop very swollen udders just before kidding. If the udder is of normal temperature and contains no abnormal

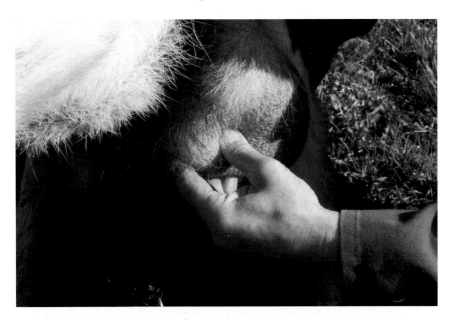

PLATE 6.11 Oedema of the udder. Applying thumb pressure

hardness then oedema is most probably present. To test for this, press the thumb into the skin and if a depression or pit remains, then oedema (or fluid) is present in the udder. This is a natural phenomenon and is normally of no significance. If the doe is in great pain when it comes to milking her, then massaging may help.

Should the problem persist your veterinary surgeon may prescribe an injection to remove some of this fluid. Normally the fluid will pass away in time.

One study has described a method of incising the skin to release the fluid. I would never resort to such treatment and I certainly would not suggest that goatkeepers try it.

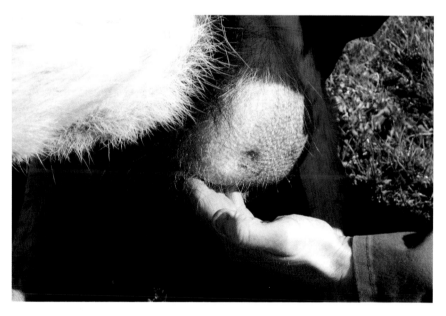

PLATE 6.12   Oedema of the udder. 'Pit' left after pressure by thumb

BLOOD IN THE MILK

This occurs from time to time, the milker noticing pink milk. It usually follows a blow to the udder. In newly kidded does this finding is more frequently a symptom of a ruptured blood capillary. At kidding the udder becomes congested and with a build-up of pressure of milk, small blood vessels occasionally burst. The blood leaks into the milk, turning it pink. Normally the vessels cease bleeding within a short time, heal up and no more is seen. The milk is aesthetically unpleasant and must not be sold. Assuming that no mastitis is present, it could safely be fed to dogs and cats. If the haemorrhage is very severe, call your veterinary surgeon and he will give injections to arrest the haemorrhage.

Fall in Milk Yield

This is a common symptom of many diseases, especially ones that make the doe go off her food. It cannot be considered alone and as it is an important symptom, you must seek professional help from your vet. If it affects the whole herd, before seeking help check the obvious points, such as whether the water supply is functioning.

Goatpox (Capripox)

Two types of goatpox occur, a mild form and a very severe (malignant) form (Capripox virus). The malignant form is not present in the United Kingdom or North America but affects goats in Africa and Asia (see page 17). Benign goatpox causes raised papules and pustules on the skin of the udder and teats. It can also affect the lips and mouth. The pox may persist for five or six weeks, gradually becoming 'crusty' as time passes.

Treatment
Applying ointment to the sores may help to reduce spread and also encourage rapid healing. There are many suitable udder creams available which contain an antiseptic such as cetrimide or chlorhexidine. The ointment should be removed by wiping all the teats with a disposable towel, before milking. Affected goats should be milked last and the equipment sterilised in order to attempt to reduce the spread of pox. Having said this, in large herds, one is often obliged to live with the problem.

MALE MILKERS

Occasionally bucks may commence to produce milk and mastitis may even occur in the 'udder'. (*See* page 149.)

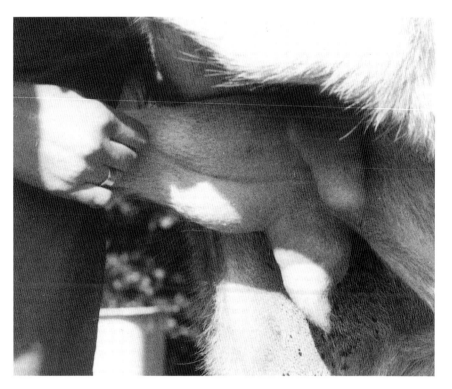

PLATE 6.13   Buck with glands producing milk

SUPERNUMERARY TEATS

Some kids are born with more than two teats. The British Goat Society rightly discourages goatkeepers from breeding from goats affected by this condition. From a breeding point of view these kids are best culled or sold for meat, in order to prevent the problem being passed on to the next generation.

If the decision is made to remove the teats then this is best done at a young age so that no scars remain when the doe comes into milk. They can be surgically snipped off using curved scissors and the wound dressed with antiseptic powder or cream. Discuss this with your vet.

DEFORMED TEATS

Various teat abnormalities have been recorded in goats, including 'fish tail teats'. They should be assumed to be inherited conditions, and the goats should not be bred from. Check breeding females as young as possible to avoid rearing goats with abnormal teats.

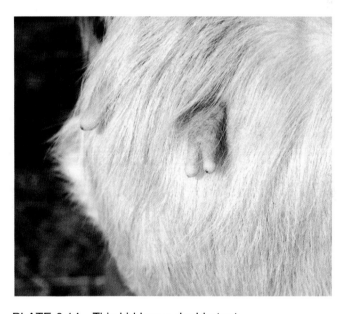

PLATE 6.14   This kid has a double teat

BLIND UDDERS

Occasionally does will kid and produce an udder one side of which will not milk, even though the milk-secreting tissue is present. The problem stems from a milk duct that is not open.

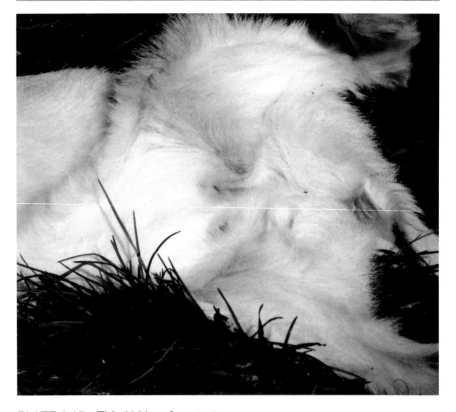

PLATE 6.15   This kid has four teats

Reports indicate that the condition is inherited. Sometimes careful surgery will enable the teat to be opened up to allow milking of the half. Any such interference, however, carries with it a risk of mastitis developing. These goats should not be bred from.

WARTS ON TEATS

Warts are benign tumours of the skin. Frequently they are associated with a virus. Generally they disappear after several months as immunity develops. (*See* page 251.)

Teat Sores

Sores develop on teats for various reasons, for example following chapping, when teats remain wet in cold weather. Treat them quickly with cream such as Dermisol (Pfizer), because they are reservoirs for mastitis organisms.

Staphylococcal Dermatitis

A frequently unresponsive and difficult skin infection, often involving the udder, is caused by the staphylococcal germ. Creams and even injections of antibiotics often fail to eliminate it. This is probably because the goat's immune mechanism is poor. Probably the best results are obtained by using an autogenous vaccine, which is prepared from the pustules and re-injected into the goat. Discuss the matter with your vet.

Chapter 7

PROBLEMS ASSOCIATED WITH BREEDING, PREGNANCY AND BIRTH

BREEDING

SEASON

In northern latitudes goats are seasonal breeders, only capable of mating at certain times of the year. In the tropics does come on heat all the year round. In the United Kingdom the season extends from September to February. Conversely in the southern hemisphere the season occurs from March to August.

THE REPRODUCTIVE CYCLE

Several hormones are involved in the delicate functioning of the oestrous cycle. They are listed below with their abbreviations and their sites of production.

Hormone	Abbreviation	Site of production
Follicle stimulating hormone	FSH	Anterior pituitary
Oestrogen	—	Follicle in ovary
Luteinising hormone	LH	Anterior pituitary
Progesterone	—	Corpus luteum in ovary
Prostaglandin	PG	Uterus

At the start of the breeding season the cycle proceeds as illustrated in Figure 7.1.

172

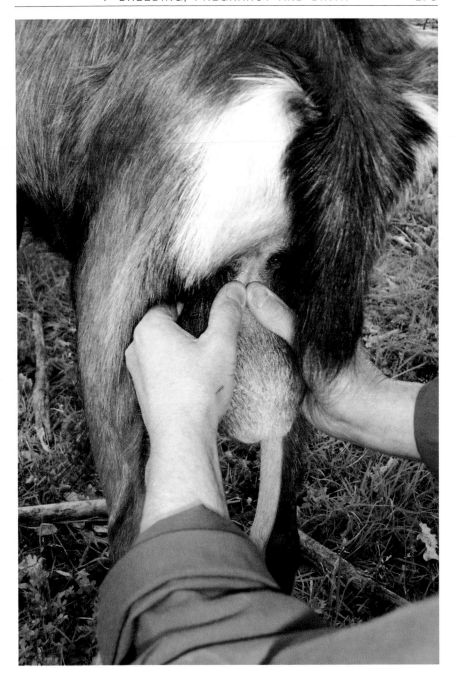

PLATE 7.1 Check the buck's testicles well in advance of the breeding season

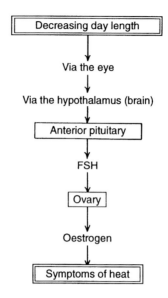

FIGURE 7.1   Chain of events leading to oestrus

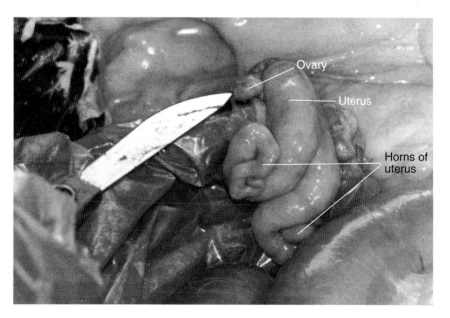

PLATE 7.2   The uterus and ovaries of a non-pregnant doe; the knife point
is on one ovary

The stimulus of decreasing day length causes the release of follicle stimulating hormone from the anterior pituitary. This causes the development of follicles in the ovary. The follicles then release oestrogens which result in the doe exhibiting the symptoms of oestrus or heat. The circulating oestrogen acts upon the hypothalamus/pituitary to reduce FSH and to stimulate the production of LH. This results in ovulation and an egg is released from the now mature follicle in the ovary. A summary of this process is given in Figure 7.2.

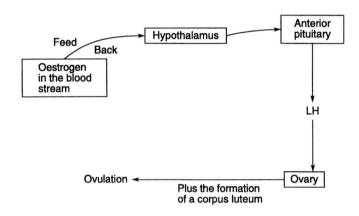

FIGURE 7.2   The hormonal action leading to ovulation

The corpus luteum forms from what remains of the follicle after ovulation. This starts to produce progesterone which is necessary to maintain pregnancy. All this takes place in about one week, commencing a few days before the heat is noticed. If pregnancy does not interrupt the cycle, then prostaglandin is released from the uterus. This hormone is 'luteolytic' and causes the corpus luteum to disappear. Once this is gone so too is the progesterone and the whole cycle starts once again. Should pregnancy result during the cycle then prostaglandin is not released and the corpus luteum remains.

Signs of Heat (Oestrus)
Does on heat become vocal, calling loudly. The vulva swells slightly and a clear mucus discharge may be noticed. A great deal of tail wagging occurs and the area around the tail looks

characteristically 'dirty' or 'wet'. Very rarely the does may show mounting behaviour, the doe on heat being mounted by another doe. A 'teaser' buck or a nymphomaniac female can be used for the purpose of identifying goats on heat. The use of a teaser (vasectomised) buck may assist in the detection of heat in larger herds and allow specific matings to be made. A vasectomised buck is rendered infertile by cutting the tubes which carry sperm from the testes to the penis. His libido and interest in mating still remains and thus he can indicate which females are on heat. The oestrous females are then placed with a stud buck for a fertile mating.

Occasionally females with ovarian problems are retained, when they behave in a male fashion by mounting other does. Again they indicate the does on heat for the goatkeeper. Care must be taken to distinguish 'dominance' mounting, (when bossy does mount does lower down the pecking order), from does mounting because the goat underneath is on heat.

Length and Frequency of Heat
This is extremely variable. I have seen heats as short as twelve hours and as long as forty-eight. Other authors give between 36–39 hours and 13–27 hours, and one colleague reports a four-hour heat in his own doe. Within the season goats come on heat approximately every 19–21 days.

MATING

A doe in heat will normally stand to be mounted, although a nervous doe in strange surroundings may fidget and move. The mating is quick. The male mounts, penetrates and after a few thrusts throws back his head when ejaculation occurs.

ARTIFICIAL INSEMINATION (AI)

Artificial insemination is now available in the United Kingdom, Europe and North America. The frozen semen is stored in liquid nitrogen after collection. This enables selected bucks to be used to up-grade poorer quality females without much risk of disease spread. This may promise an easy alternative for goatkeepers who live a great distance from the buck of their choice.

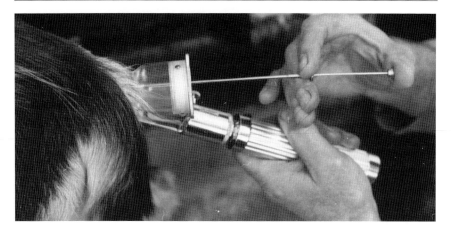

PLATE 7.3   Artificial insemination. The speculum allows the operator to locate the cervix

EXTENDING THE BREEDING SEASON

There are three methods of advancing the breeding season:

1. Using light
2. Using melatonin implants
3. Using vaginal sponges.

Sometimes a combination of methods is used depending upon the circumstances.

Advancing the breeding season by light treatment

The trigger to the sexual activity of goats is the change in day length, which is transmitted by the eye to the brain. Specifically, in Northern latitudes it is the decreasing hours of daylight in autumn. There is a chain of events leading to hormone release that initiates the sexual cycles. Figure 7.3 illustrates this.

Using artificial light one can create short days after a period of long days and 'shift' the breeding season to commence in spring or early summer. For example, if one has artificially 'long' days in winter, one can then reduce that light, (after a minimum of 75 days) and begin to shorten the daylength (mimic autumn). This results in the goats coming on heat in the spring hence kidding in the autumn and thus producing winter milk.

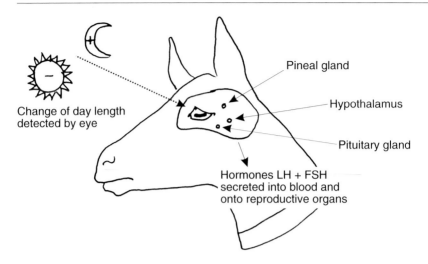

FIGURE 7.3   The effect of light on reproduction

Research has revealed that there is a 'photo-receptive period' in the day which occurs 16 to 17 hours after dawn. If sufficient light is supplied at this time it is equivalent to a 'long' day of summer. Thus, for goats continually in a building in winter and spring one can commence a day with artificial light at 6 a.m.

The goats are given three hours light until the natural daylight is sufficient. More artificial light is then supplied 16 hours after the artificial dawn for a period of two hours. That light is given from 21 to 23.00 hours. This protocol must be started before mid-March and sufficient light must be supplied.

If natural mating is used (as opposed to artificial insemination) then the bucks must undergo the same light treatment. The sexes can be together in the same building for these 'long' days. The bucks are best removed after that, when the 'short days'

Dec	Dec	Jan	Jan	Feb	15 to Feb 28	Mar	15 Mar to 31	April	April	May	May
Light	light	light	light	light							
							Bucks in				

FIGURE 7.4   Diagram of light treatment protocol

commence, in order to improve the sudden 'buck effect', when they are put back in with the females just prior to breeding.

More details on this technique can be obtained from: technipel@inst-elevage.asso.fr

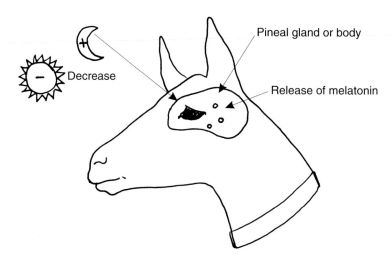

Decrease

Pineal gland or body

Release of melatonin

FIGURE 7.5 The effect of light on melatonin secretion

Using melatonin to advance the breeding cycle

Figure 7.5 shows that melatonin is secreted by the pineal body. It is only secreted at night.

Melatonin is the intermediary between the pineal body and the hypothalamus which initiates sexual cycles. Greater quantities of melatonin are secreted on long nights and this is the stimulus for the onset of reproductive cycles in the autumn in the northern hemisphere.

By implanting a long release depot of melatonin (Melovine .CEVA) under the skin of the goat, one is able to mimic the onset of winter and hence start the reproductive cycles.

PROTOCOL

The bucks and females are separated a week before the implant is made. For the bucks, three 18 mg implants are given. A week later just one 18 mg implant is administered to the does. The bucks are then re-introduced 6 to 7 weeks later and mating commences within a short period.

This technique can be used following light treatment to mimic long days. (*See* previous section, THE EFFECT OF LIGHT ON REPRODUCTION.) It is recommended that the melatonin treatment is started after mid-March in France. Readers should seek further information from the manufacturers of melatonin for precise details of usage.

3. The use of vaginal sponges
The constraints of the natural breeding season can be partially overcome by artificially bringing does into heat using sponges. This is best attempted in the months just before the season normally commences. Thus, July or August may be suitable in the United Kingdom, early June in continental Europe, and June to August in North America. In the southern hemisphere, for equivalent latitudes, December, January and February could be considered suitable. The advantages of doing this are to have does kidding early on in the year. This extends the time during which milk is produced in quantity. In many countries the price paid for 'winter' milk is also higher and thus the enterprise becomes more profitable.

Procedure
1. Progesterone-impregnated sponges are carefully inserted into the vagina of the doe using an antiseptic cream to prevent the introduction of infection (Veramix sponges containing 60 mg of medroxyprogesterone or Chronogest [Intervet] are suitable). It may be easier to insert them using a clean, well-lubricated finger, rather than the applicator. This is especially true in maiden females. The sponge should be positioned about halfway along the vagina, not too close to the cervix.
2. 500 IU of PMSG (pregnant mare serum gonadotrophin) are injected 10 to 12 days later, together with an injection of prostaglandin (in separate syringes).
3. The sponges are withdrawn 12–14 days after insertion (they have a little 'tail' of nylon cord by which they can be pulled out). Other goats will sometimes nibble the cord and pull the sponge out by accident.
4. Heat should occur 12–36 hours after the sponge is withdrawn.
5. Natural service or artificial insemination of the doe in heat can then take place.

Results

The success rate for this technique is generally in the order of over 50 per cent pregnancies. The nearer to the natural breeding season that this technique is carried out, the greater is the success rate. It is difficult to determine which does have conceived because the non-pregnant does resume seasonal anoestrus. They do not come on heat until the normal breeding season has commenced. The goats can be scanned to check the success rate if a suitable scanner operator can be found. If no pregnancy results the goatkeeper has lost little and the doe is served, as normal, when she is on heat. One practical drawback of this technique is that the sponges come in packs of fifty. Your veterinary surgeon may be prepared to split up packs and insert sponges into individual does in the smaller herd. The technique should not be attempted less than 170 days after kidding, because the lactation will reduce chances of success.

Use of sponges in goats in France

French commercial research underlines the benefit to be obtained from 'grouping' milking goats in order to increase yield. This means bringing groups of goats into heat at the same time in order to kid them at the same time. Sponges are used to bring about this effect. The benefits gained from 'grouping' does and producing heat before the normal breeding season are many. They include; more milk, a shorter kidding interval, a longer lactation and less barren goats. It should be noted that only poor results are gained from goatlings.

For Young Goats (Sponges)

Only goats >7 months or >30 kg.
1. Sponge day minus 10, rupture hymen with finger inserted into vagina.
2. Day 0 insert sponge (lamb type).
3. Day 0 plus 9   <15 June   >15 June
  inject PMSG   300 IU   250 IU
    Cloprostenol   100 mg   100 mg
4. Day 0 plus 11 sponge out.
5. Day 0 plus 13 insemination (48 hours after sponge removed).

Some Practical Considerations of Sponging

The technique, though very useful, is far from perfect and the success rate of bringing goats into heat very variable. When

	DAY	D 0		D 9	D 10	D11	D12	D13
SAANEN BEFORE 15 JUNE	MORNING			PMSG + CP 9 h		REMOVE 9 h		AI₂ 9 h (±2 h)
	AFTER NOON						AI₁ 14 h (+ 2 h)	
SAANEN AFTER 15 JUNE	MORNING	SPONGE INSERTED				SPONGE		AI 11 h (±2 h)
	AFTER NOON			PMSG + CP 14 h		REMOVE 14 h		
FRENCH ALPINE	MORNING					REMOVE		
	AFTER NOON			PMSG + CP 14 h		REMOVE 14 h		AI 9 h (±2 h)

THE DOSE OF PMSG DEPENDS UPON THE MILK YIELD

CP : Prostaglandin (Cloprostenol)

(N.B. : Removing the sponge in the morning increases fertility)

YIELD	BEFORE 15/06	AFTER 16/06
>3.5 kg/l	600 IU	500 IU
<3.5 kg/l	500 IU	400 IU

Different procedures are adopted for the goats sponged before and after 15 June. The explanation is that it is harder to bring goats into heat before that date than after it.

D0 means day zero and is the day of sponge insertion.
D9 means day 9 and so on.

Much research has gone into the subject and the exact timing is important even to the hour indicated for the injections etc.

AI_1 means first insemination
AI_2 means second insemination.

The bottom table indicates how higher yielding does require slightly higher hormone doses in order to achieve the same results.

FIGURE 7.6   French recommendations for the use of sponges in previously bred goats

inserting the sponge, if an antiseptic cream is not supplied, spray the sponge with an antibiotic aerosol before insertion. Otherwise there is a high percentage of nasty smelling infected sponges on removal. If the technique is used for several years running on the same goats, a high proportion of them become 'refractory' to the technique and it doesn't work. Ensure that there is enough 'buck power' available when the sponges are withdrawn because many goats are on heat together. Practical experience reveals that not only the sponged individuals come on heat, but it tends to set off a large group of females in the herd in a 'copy cat' manner. Goatkeepers wishing to advance their breeding season may well find this trick useful. Sponge a few goats and the rest of the herd will probably follow suit in a fairly short time. This brings forward the kiddings and has the added advantage of 'grouping' them.

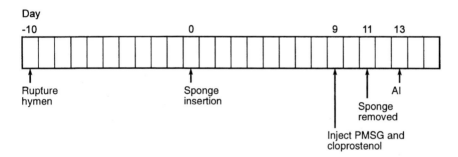

FIGURE 7.7   Use of sponges in unbred goats older than 7 months or heavier than 30 kg

IDENTIFYING BREEDING AND MATING PROBLEMS

The broad types of problems that may present themselves are listed below. Having identified the type of abnormality, the reader can refer to the relevant section in order to try and determine the cause.

1. Does that fail to come on heat
2. Unmated does that come on heat and then cease to cycle
3. Does with heats of irregular length
4. Does with regular heats after mating (repeat breeders)

5. Physical problems of mating
6. Further investigation of infertility in does
7. Infertility due to intersex.

1. Does that Fail to Come on Heat

Three important questions should be posed before complex investigations are initiated. The most important question to ask oneself is, of course, is there a problem? Could the heats be occurring without being noticed? Heats may persist for very short periods of even just a few hours. Is it possible that she is pregnant? This is especially relevant if the doe has been brought in from elsewhere. It may well be worth getting her scanned before taking any further action.

Is the goat an intersex? This is only likely in a maiden goat. Such animals are always infertile (*see* INFERTILITY DUE TO INTERSEX, page 187).

Non-lactating does that fail to come on heat

Failure of does to come on heat, between, say October and November, must be treated as a problem. Often the trouble is that the doe is either too thin or too fat.

Goats in poor bodily condition may be undernourished. In these instances increase the total food ration, especially of energy food such as cereals. Observe whether cycles commence and if they do not, ask your veterinary surgeon for advice. The first step would probably be to sponge the goat. If that fails he will probably give the doe an injection of prostaglandin to bring her into heat. One and a half ml of Lutalyse (7.5 mg) PGF_2 will normally stimulate oestrus within a few days; 0.5 ml of Estrumate (Coopers) is reported to be equally effective. This treatment often works because the doe was having 'silent' or inapparent heats. If some underlying disease is responsible for the goat's condition, your veterinary surgeon will advise you on this.

On the other hand, excessive fatness may affect a goat's cycles. Slim the goat down and seek your vet's advice; an injection of prostaglandin will possibly bring her into heat. After she has been mated try to get her into lean condition, otherwise she will be too fat at kidding.

Milking does that fail to come on heat

Does kidded for less than 4 months come on heat while they are still milking but the lactation may suppress the oestrus (in the first part of lactation). If the doe has kidded within the previous

4 months, leave her alone and wait to see if heats recur naturally.

Does advanced in lactation that are milking well may fail to come into heat if their diet is poor. Increase the energy food intake of these does for 3 weeks. If no heat occurs, consult your vet who will probably bring the heat on by an injection of prostaglandin. Sponges are an alternative.

2. Unmated Does that Come on Heat and then Cease to Cycle

In my experience, these goats can often be made to start cycling again by using prostaglandin injections, providing that it is not too late in the season (i.e. before February).

The cause may be either movement to new surroundings or silent heats.

3. Does with Cycles of Irregular Length

Goats show a wide variation in length of the oestrous cycle. Different authors quote varying lengths; for example three sources quote the following:

17–23 days
18–21 days
19–21 days

It is probably safe to assume that anything outside the 17–23 days is abnormal.

Short cycles or continuous heat

At the beginning of the breeding season some goats come on heat twice within a week; they then settle down to normal-length cycles. Some does exhibit frequent heat periods or they appear to be in a continuous state of heat. This is normally an ovarian problem where cysts develop in the ovary. It is as if the ovary becomes 'stuck' in the heat phase of the cycle; oestrogens are produced and they are responsible for the signs of heat.

The condition can be treated, unless the symptoms have progressed to the stage of masculinisation, when the doe begins to behave as if she were a buck. In these cases the animal is best slaughtered. Some goatkeepers with large herds retain these masculinised animals because they can be usefully employed to indicate other does that are on heat. (*See* Nymphomaniac Female page 176.)

Hormones can be given by your vet to change the state of the ovary. He would probably use chorionic gonadotrophin (Chorulon Injection, Intervet Laboratories Ltd).

This formulation substitutes the luteinising hormone secreted by the anterior pituitary gland. The chorionic gonadotrophin promotes maturation of the follicle, ovulation and the formation of a Corpus Luteum. Previously this product was licensed for use in goats and the dose rate was 1,000 i.u.

This condition is fairly common; for example in one study of dead goats at abattoirs, 24 cases were seen in a total of 1,020 goats. It must be remembered, however, that some of these goats may well have been slaughtered because of this condition; thus it may have been a biased sample.

Long cycles

Occasionally, long cycles may be detected in does. If they are multiples of 20 days, e.g. 40 days, then it is possible that they are in fact normal cycles and the owner has missed observing a heat period. In other cases early embryonic death may have occurred; that is, the doe conceived to service, but the embryo died. In this case the doe might go for some time before she has her next heat. Discuss this with your vet if you have a problem.

4. Does with Regular Heats After Mating (Repeat Breeders)

There are a number of reasons why a doe may return to service at regular intervals after being served:

- The buck may be infertile. This can normally be checked by finding out if other does served by him have conceived. It is also possible to check a sample of his semen in order to clarify the situation. Use another buck.
- Does can show heat during a pregnancy. The signs of oestrus are usually less well defined. If in doubt have the doe served, it should normally do no harm.
- If the doe is milking then this may be detrimental to her conceiving (high yielders). This is very rare because normally the peak of lactation (three to four weeks after kidding) is in the spring or early summer. As the breeding season is in the autumn, unless induced artificially, the doe should be well on in lactation. Theoretically it is a stress on the doe to support an embryo and to carry on yielding a great deal of milk. If this is suspected, increasing the energy ration at service may help to get the doe to conceive.
- The service is being carried out at the wrong time. Possibly too early on in the heat period.

- Dietary insufficiency. Start a course of proprietary goat or cow dairy ration, known to include minerals and vitamins.
- Infections and adhesions around the reproductive tract. Seek veterinary advice.

5. Physical Problems of Mating

Occasionally, everything is theoretically right in that the doe is on heat, the buck is with her but successful mating does not occur. The majority of problems in this situation would lie with the male.

The buck

Reluctance to serve may be due to painful hind legs and feet. Arthritis seems to be a fairly common problem of stud bucks. It is probably caused by excessive feeding of calcium and keeping them on cold, damp, bedding. Lameness from other causes should also be considered. (*See* Chapters 3 and 8.)

Overwork: only when severely underfed and undernourished, will a buck refuse to mount, but attention should be given to the buck's nutrition. During the breeding season bucks often go off their food and it may be useful to vary the diet in order to try to tempt them to eat. Some young inexperienced bucks may fail to mate, if so try them with a quiet experienced female when she is overtly on heat.

6. Further Investigation of Infertility in Does

Modern technology such as scanning and the use of laproscopy has meant that sophisticated examinations can now be made on infertile does. These can reveal, for example, adhesions around the ovaries and fallopian tubes. From abattoir surveys, such problems around the reproductive tracts, can be quite common. They can give rise to symptoms of infertility, often because the eggs fail to reach the uterus.

7. Infertility Due to Intersex

Kids may be born which have a mixture of male and female genitalia. For example they may be predominantly male-like, having testicles but no penis. Instead they have a slit-like vulva and uterine horns. These kids are, of course, normally culled. Sometimes, these anatomical problems are not very apparent, the kids are reared and the first sign of a problem is when they have breeding problems.

The progeny of polled (naturally hornless) goats are frequently infertile. It is therefore best not to rear these animals for breeding purposes. As a prevention policy always mate goats which are polled or of unknown status to a horned goat.

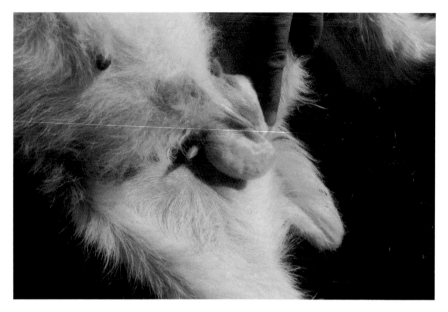

PLATE 7.4   Hermaphrodite

8. The Cryptorchid

A buck could have either one (hemi-cryptorchid) or possibly both testicles (cryptorchid) retained in the abdomen. This can lead to poor sperm production and infertility. In adult goats the testicles are very obvious but it is important to check young kids which are destined to become breeding animals. Ensure that both testicles have descended into the scrotum.

PREGNANCY AND KIDDING

The average length of pregnancy is 150 days but there is obviously some variation around this mean. It is not abnormal for goats to kid four days either side of 150 days. Breed differences account for some of the variations.

TESTS FOR PREGNANCY

The goatkeeper will find it useful to know whether or not the doe has conceived. Several different methods are available and these are described below.

Absence of heats

In many species such as the cow, the fact that the served cow does not come on heat again is a fairly good indication of pregnancy. Alas, some goats do exhibit heat symptoms during pregnancy and therefore this indication, although useful, is not fool-proof. Does with a 'cloudburst' (pseudo-pregnancy) do not come on heat either (*see* CLOUDBURST, page 195).

The milk test

Laboratories will carry out a test on the milk of a lactating goat in order to test for pregnancy. Formerly, the progesterone test was used at twenty-four days but this gives rise to an unacceptable number of false positives. The present test can only be performed at fifty days and it involves the demonstration of oestrone sulphate. Occasionally, after having a positive test, something may

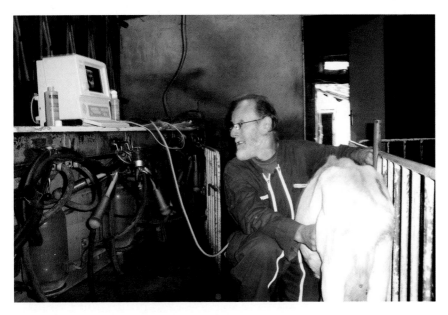

PLATE 7.5   Use of a scanner for pregnancy diagnosis

happen to the foetus late on in pregnancy so that no kid is born. The drawback of this test is that the doe must be milking and it cannot, therefore, be used on goatlings in-kid for the first time.

Real-time scanning
This technique is now used commonly in many countries. It is available in the United Kingdom for sheep flocks and for goats also. Its value lies in being able to differentiate single and multiple foetuses. Cloudbursts can also be detected earlier by the scan. This is the method of choice in countries where it is available.

The rectal pole technique
Originally designed for sheep, this test can be applied to goats and Guss (*see* References) recommends its use in does between 70 and 110 days of pregnancy. In essence the pole is inserted into the rectum in order to allow the examiner to feel the pregnant uterus more easily. The examination would seem to cause some stress to the doe. Modern techniques such as scanning makes this method redundant in developed countries.

X-ray determination
This technique can be used to identify the bones of the kids in the uterus. It is little used on account of the time and expense involved.

Conclusion
Scanning is the most reliable of all these methods but it does require sophisticated equipment. It is non-invasive, carried out with the doe standing normally.

PROBLEMS ARISING DURING PREGNANCY

ABORTION

Abortion can occur for one of many reasons including infections, vitamin A deficiency or pregnancy toxaemia. The number of abortions that occur in the United Kingdom is probably fairly small, based upon the VIDA II records for a period of eight years (Defra). The types of abortion experienced in different countries can vary tremendously. The different kinds of infection that can be associated with abortion in goats are numerous and they include:

- Enzootic abortion (chlamydia – *C. psittaci*)
- Toxoplasma spp
- Salmonella spp
- Mycoplasma
- Vibrio (Campylobacter)
- Q-fever (*Coxiella burnetii*)
- Paratuberculosis (Johne's disease)
- Listeria monocytogenes
- Brucella abortus
- Brucella melitensis.

Procedure if Abortion Occurs

Isolate the doe, keep the placenta and aborted foetus in a polythene bag. As a precaution, clean up and burn the material from where the abortion occurred, in case it was an infectious cause. Exclude other goats from the area. Now one must decide how to proceed. This depends upon the size of your herd and how cautious you are. If in doubt discuss the matter with your vet. As some abortions will always occur from non-infectious causes, one has to wait and see if one has a significant problem, or if the abortion is an isolated incident. One solution is to deep-freeze your specimens, keep the doe isolated, and carefully monitor the situation. If another doe aborts, get both the samples off to your vet as soon as possible. Your vet will probably send samples to a laboratory for examination and the more of the placenta and foetus you keep, the better the chance of determining the cause. A blood sample from the doe will be required for many investigations. The percentage of examinations which reveal an infectious cause is fairly small but this is partly due to the fact that laboratories do not always receive the correct samples. **Note** that some agents that cause abortion are responsible for **disease in human beings**, so observe personal hygiene – wear gloves. Pregnant women are strongly advised to avoid this area of work.

Confirmed Infectious Abortions

What can be done following diagnosed abortions in a herd depends upon what organism was involved. In some instances, it is best to mix all kidded or non-pregnant does with the aborted doe in order to try and *spread* the infection! The reason being that if the goats are infected while they are not pregnant, no disease will result but they will become immune and will not abort the following year. This policy should be adopted with chlamydial abortion (EAE). With listeria and salmonella abortion one should strive to prevent the spread of infection. Your veterinary surgeon will advise you on this complex subject. One must remember that many of these infections cause abortion in sheep and goats and therefore when the species are run together, the risk of abortion may be higher. Incidentally, rams will mate with does but the foetus is aborted.

Chlamydiosis

If this infection is diagnosed in the aborted material, then the rest of the herd must be considered. It is important to understand that the agent causes no disease in non-pregnant animals. Any unbred (non pregnant) does should be put in contact with the aborted animals. This spreads the disease, and thus the immunity around the herd. It would be wise to inject any other pregnant does with tetracyclines by the intramuscular route to try to prevent them from aborting. Your vet will guide you on this. In future years, control will rely upon vaccination of the young, unbred does (Enzovax, Intervet UK Ltd). (*See* 'Before Mating', page 215.) Although the vaccine is not licensed for use in goats in the UK, it is used. The aborted does and the in-contact females will be immune and require no vaccine. Vaccination of the replacement females can start at five months and must be completed four weeks prior to mating. This enables them to develop immunity before they become pregnant. Do not vaccinate pregnant females.

Toxoplasmosis

A coccidium of cats, *T. gondii* is responsible for this disease and it affects most mammals, including goats and humans. In goats, early embryonic death, abortion, stillbirth and weak kids are recognised indicators of infection. The range of these indicators depends upon the stage at which the pregnant goat was exposed to infection. Young cats excrete the oocysts for a fairly short period after they are contaminated. They pick up the parasite by eating vermin. The faeces of the infected cats contain the oocysts. Cats then contaminate goat feed which in turn infects the goats. Attempting to reduce exposure to young cats may help; however, this may lead to increased vermin such as rats, which carry other diseases.

If a goat aborts due to this disease then she should be isolated from the other goats until they have all kidded.

Diagnosis of the disease is by laboratory examination of the aborted foetus. Blood samples from aborted goats are also useful in confirming the involvement of Toxoplasmosis.

Recently a vaccine has been produced to control toxoplasmosis in sheep (Intervet). It may be used in goats although it is not actually licensed for use in the goat. The vaccine must not be used in pregnant animals and the milk/meat from goats vaccinated should not be consumed by humans for six weeks after the injection. It is suggested that goats should be vaccinated annually. Females can be vaccinated from five months old ideally to be completed four weeks before mating. In sheep this vaccine can be given at the same time as Enzovax (above). The injections are made at two different sites. Neither vaccine is licensed for use in goats in the UK.

Great care should be taken when handling this live vaccine. Goatkeepers would only consider using this vaccine if a serious toxoplasmosis problem was present in the flock. The administration is by intramuscular injection.

In humans toxoplasmosis causes flu-like symptoms and abortion in females.

Q Fever (Coxiellosis)

An infection of humans and animals caused by *Coxiella burnetii*. It is a zoonose, meaning that humans can catch the disease from animals or their products. Recently Q fever infection in a French hospital was traced back to patients working with goats and/or consuming goat products. The germ was isolated in the goats' milk. The symptoms of the disease in humans include fever, weakness and headaches.

Occurrence
It affects many species of domesticated and wild animals. It can be found in urine, milk and uterine discharges.

Symptoms
Late abortion is the main symptom in goats. In a newly infected herd the number of goats aborting may be 100 per cent. In later years the developing immunity reduces this figure.

Diagnosis
Diagnostic confirmation is made either direct from smears made
from the aborted material or from blood tests on pregnant goats.
The most common blood test is the CFT where a titre is considered to indicate infection.

Prevention
Vaccines are available in some countries such as France, where
the disease is very prevalent. In some regions of France this
cause of abortion is the most frequently diagnosed infection.

Public health
Wear disposable gloves when dealing with aborted materials.
Goats milk from affected herds should be heat treated before con-
sumption by humans.

BRUCELLOSIS

Brucella organisms infect an animal's placenta and udder, causing
abortion and mastitis. A great deal of misunderstanding arises
among goatkeepers on this topic, mainly stemming from the difference between the words 'possibility' and 'probability'. Perhaps
I can clarify the situation.

Two strains of this organism infect goats, both of which can
cause disease in humans; they are *Brucella melitensis* and
Brucella abortus. In humans, they cause Malta fever and undu-
lant fever respectively. *Brucella melitensis* is widespread in goats
throughout the world but has never been recorded in the United
Kingdom.

Brucella abortus, which is a disease of cattle, can occasionally
affect goats.[*] Having stated that it does affect goats, one must add
that infection is extremely unlikely. The possibility of it causing
problems in the United Kingdom in the future is even more
remote because the disease has now been eradicated from cattle.
This is true of many parts of the world where successful control
schemes for cattle have been implemented; for example, in the
USA, Australia, New Zealand and most of Europe. However,
goatkeepers should always be aware that brucellosis can be
transmitted to humans by way of an infected animal's milk.

Brucella melitensis is a bacterial disease which can affect most

---

[*] See MATHUS, T. N. (1967) *Indian Journal of Veterinary Science, 37*, 272–86.

species of domestic animal, although sheep and goats, particularly milking breeds, are the most susceptible. Cattle may occasionally be affected and the disease may also appear in pigs. In humans the disease is known as Malta fever, and is similar to, and perhaps more severe than, that caused by *B. abortus*. Strict hygiene precautions should be followed when handling animals or aborted foetuses. The UK, Ireland and many European countries are free from this disease.

Symptoms
Infection is normally through inhalation or skin wounds: transmission between species occurs readily. Humans usually become infected by ingestion of affected milk. The post-kidding discharges (after-birth) of infected does contain large numbers of bacteria whether or not the animal has aborted. After abortion, infection may persist in the uterus for many months, and in the udder for years. Viable kids from infected females may also be infected but show negative blood tests, they may discharge infection following their first kidding or abortion. These animals would thus be a significant risk when imported into an uninfected herd so it is essential that animals be added only from herds of known free status.

When infection is first introduced into a flock or herd, there may be an 'abortion storm'. Fever, depression, mastitis, arthritis, testicular infection or nervous signs may accompany acute infection. A chronically infected herd may show few abortions or clinical signs due to the partial immunity developed over years.

Estimating the Age of the Aborted Kid
Sometimes it is useful to know at what stage of pregnancy the abortion occurred. This can be estimated from the size of the aborted kid. The following information may be of help:

length of foetus at 30 days: 1.4 cm
length of foetus at 145 days: 43.0 cm

The eyes open between the 130th and 140th day of pregnancy.

CLOUDBURST (PSEUDOPREGNANCY, FALSE PREGNANCY)

Reports, surveys and personal experience indicate that this condition is quite commonly seen in goats in the United Kingdom. Why the condition occurs is unknown. An abattoir survey in

Scandinavia revealed three cases out of 1,020 goats. Two Indian surveys of a similar scale recorded a low frequency. By contrast, the author noted two cases in a much smaller sample of goat (231) in the United Kingdom. A thorough and large scale study of 10,000 French goats was carried out in 1989–1990. The findings were that 50 per cent of the farms experienced the condition and by scanning the goats, that one out of ten farms had more than 5 per cent of animals affected. In the two year study the prevalence was 2.1 per cent and 2.9 per cent of all the goats scanned.

It must be said that the French work was dealing with a large proportion of goats that had been sponged, their season brought forward, and grouped together.

Symptoms
Due to the influence of the ovarian hormone, progesterone, the doe's body becomes mistakenly convinced that it is pregnant. The signs and behaviour of pregnancy are seen and the goat can go to full term. At the time when kidding would have occurred the contents of the uterus (litres of fluid) are expelled, but no kid! Following the 'cloudburst' the doe may start to milk and have a reasonable lactation yield. Such does can be mated in subsequent years, can conceive and can even have a normal pregnancy.

One practical point to note is that cloudburst can be confirmed by the milk test or scanning. Thus, if diagnosed during pseudo pregnancy the condition can be terminated by your veterinary surgeon. This may enable the goatkeeper to have the doe served again that season and perhaps result in a normal pregnancy. The condition can occur in goats that have been sponged to advance the season, but after the kidding has occurred and before the next mating. This situation is obviously artificial and would only occur in the herds where sponging is practised.

PREGNANCY TOXAEMIA

(*See* Chapter 4, page 84.)

PROLAPSED VAGINA

The condition where the vagina of the pregnant doe starts to fall out through the vulva is seen occasionally. It is of little significance in itself but the doe may begin to strain as a natural reflex, and this is harmful. The delicate tissues also become prone to damage on hard objects and then bleed. (*See* photo, page 276.)

The replacement of the vagina is a fairly simple job for your veterinary surgeon. He may either suture the sides of the vulva to prevent prolapse, or insert a plastic retainer sold for use in sheep. The condition is thought to be due to excessive abdominal pressure and is most likely to occur in overfat does. Just before kidding, the sutures or retainer should be removed.

Prevention
Prevention relies upon keeping does lean in the early part of pregnancy.

PREPARING THE DOE FOR KIDDING

The doe in early pregnancy does not require too much food. Flushing, i.e. feeding a greater quantity of food just around mating, is sensible in order to produce a greater chance of conception. For the first three months of pregnancy the doe requires little more than maintenance, because the developing kid is only very tiny.

What happens after three months depends upon how many kids she is carrying. If the number is known, as a result of a scan, then concentrates need only be fed if she is carrying more than a singleton. This assumes a good quality forage diet. Concentrates are then fed to does carrying multiple kids, more to dams with triplets than twins, 0.5 kg maximum. If the number of kids is unknown then one has to anticipate twins and feed some concentrate. It is impossible to give accurate guidance on this because it will depend upon the quality of the forage, the number of kids and the type of concentrate.

THE KIDDING

Kiddings taking place outside at pasture, in good weather, give excellent results.

In some situations it is probably easier to kid the doe inside, especially if lights and water are available. In order that the doe acclimatises to the micro-organisms in that environment, she is best placed there about fourteen days before the birth. This will ensure that her colostral antibodies are ideal for the kid. Exercise

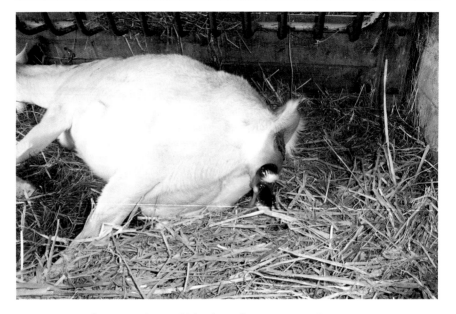

PLATE 7.6   Goat starting to kid – front feet presented

is good for her, and being out during the day is desirable. Signs of imminent kidding are a full udder, an enlarged slack vulva and restless behaviour. Most kiddings will proceed without any assistance from the owner and the best advice is to leave her alone to get on with it. Normal kiddings are over with fairly quickly, although the process can be much slower in first-time kidders.

After the water bag has appeared, discreetly check the doe every half-hour. If she strains without producing anything for longer than an hour, consult your vet. Should the doe become exhausted and the kid's feet or head be visible, then you should help her.

First of all ensure that you have clean hands, washed in plenty of soap and warm water, and wash the doe's vulva. The second step is to identify what is presented at the vulva. If two feet are showing, feel further to identify either a head or a tail. Now you know which way the kid is presented. If only legs and no head or tail can be felt ring your vet for advice. If the kid is coming backwards or forwards, then you can proceed to pull it out. The pulls should coincide with the doe's straining movements. Should you be confused about just what is presented at the vulva then do not just pull regardless because you may, for example, be pulling one leg of one kid and one leg of another. Similarly, it is easy to be confused and pull one hind leg and one fore leg and this will not come out either!

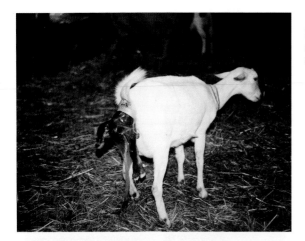

PLATE 7.7   Head and shoulders already clear of the vulva

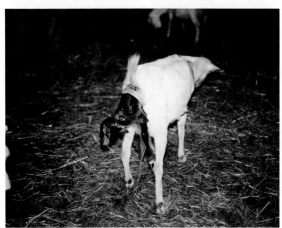

PLATE 7.8   A little more chest appears

Reviving a Weak Kid

Some kids are weak when born, especially if they were born back-feet first, and they should be assisted. Hold them upside down by the back legs and swing them gently, away from any walls or objects! This accomplishes two objectives; it clears the nostrils of any mucus or fluid and it stimulates their breathing. After swinging the kid, put your finger into the mouth to check for further mucus. Do not give up easily with a kid, many will respond if you keep stimulating them. Continue gently pumping their chests to encourage breathing and rub with straw.

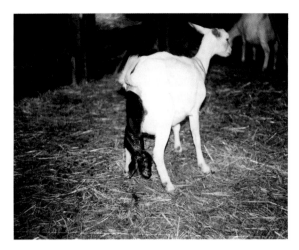

PLATE 7.9 Gravity helps the kid drop gently to the ground

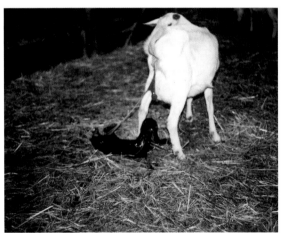

PLATE 7.10 On the ground, with the umbilical cord breaking naturally because of stretching

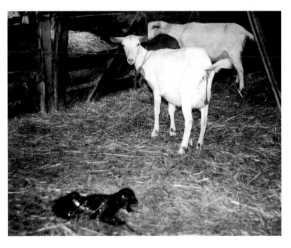

PLATE 7.11 A first time mother is not sure what happened

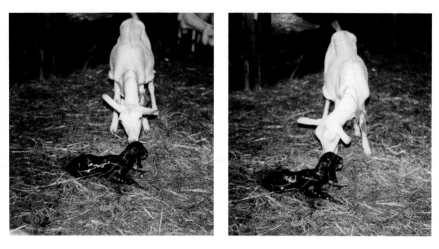

PLATE 7.12   The dam returns to investigate and then starts to lick the kid
to stimulate it.

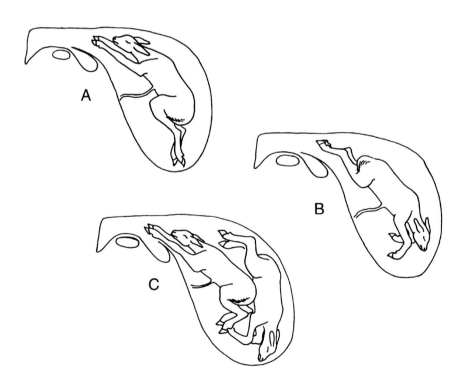

FIGURE 7.8   Normal presentations: (a) anterior; (b) posterior; (c) twins

Drugs to stimulate breathing can be given. Dopram-V (Fort Dodge) can be administered as drops under the tongue.

DIFFICULT KIDDING (DYSTOCIA)

A problem birth may arise from one of many causes. Examples are jamming of two kids at the pelvis, oversized single kids and kids awkwardly presented so that they cannot come out naturally. Some of these are illustrated in Figure 7.9.

Management of a Difficult Birth

What you do as a goatkeeper rather depends upon your experience and your aptitude. Providing that you are suitably clean and

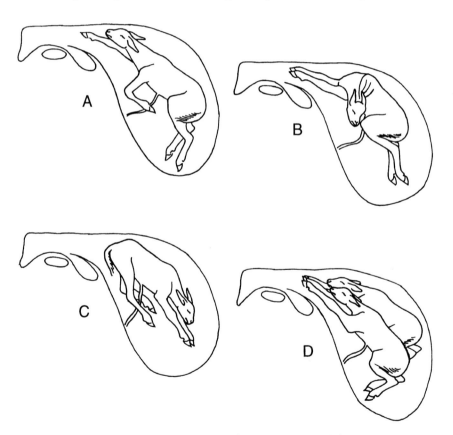

FIGURE 7.9   Abnormal presentations: (a) foreleg back; (b) head back; (c) breech; (d) twins jammed at pelvis

gentle when investigating what is going wrong inside the doe, little harm will be done. Investigation is not the same as correction and, having discovered a real problem by feeling with your hand, the best course of action may be to summon your vet. If the kid has to be repositioned this has to be done with a great deal of skill and care, so as not to rupture the uterus. If you feel that professional assistance is required, call your vet in good time so as to give him a chance to deliver live kids. The more protracted the delivery, the less the chance of live kids.

Ringwomb (failure of the cervix to dilate)

One reason for a protracted kidding is the failure of the cervix to dilate, making it impossible for the kid to be born. The doe strains but fails to produce anything at the vulva.

Recognising ringwomb

If a doe fails to produce anything after an hour of straining then she should be examined *per vaginum*. (This time guide could be extended for a first time kidder.) After a good wash in soapy water the owner may feel in to find out what is happening. Use plenty of soap as lubricant and slowly introduce the hand into the goat's vagina. If the hand and wrist can slide in easily, push further, attempting to identify a kid presented at the pelvis. If the fingers come up against the cervix no kid will be reached but the tube of the cervix identified. The 'ring' formed by the cervix will probably be open just enough to allow the operator to push two fingers through the hole.

Procedure

Frequently this problem can be overcome by a combination of drugs and patience. Drugs can be given which relax the cervix, allowing the kid to be born; an injection of prostaglandin may help. This can be assisted by gentle help using one's fingers. The fingers are inserted into the cervix and gently pulled apart in an attempt to stretch the tissue of the cervix. If this treatment fails your veterinary surgeon will probably carry out a caesarean section in order to deliver the kids.

Prevention

Do not allow does to become too fat before kidding and do encourage some exercise during pregnancy.

Torsion or Twist of the Uterus

Torsion of the uterus occurs when the whole womb and contents rotate around the axis of the cervix. This effectively seals the kids within the womb. The diagnosis is not easy for the layman and it may easily be confused with 'ring womb', described previously. If you suspect that you have a torsion of the uterus you should call your vet immediately. The correction can be made by 'rolling the doe over', whilst the uterus stays where it is – easy if you know how to do it. Once the correction has been made, the doe may deliver the kid by her own efforts. Some cases, however, will still require a caesarean section.

Oversized Kid (Foetus)

Sometimes a kid will be so large that it is impossible for it to pass through its mother's pelvis. This is especially common in very small first kidders or in goatlings served unintentionally. In such instances, after straining for over an hour, the doe will fail to produce anything at the vulva. If the goatkeeper attempts a vaginal examination with a well-lubricated hand the condition can be easily recognised. Only the fingers will be able to pass into the vagina because the bones of the pelvis will prevent the operator from going any further. Call your veterinary surgeon whose help will be required to deliver the kid by caesarean section. If the doe is worth very little one must always consider euthanasia.

Deformed Kids (Congenital Defects)

Abnormalities may be produced, such as kids with hydrocephalus (enlarged cranium), extra legs or two heads. They may be the cause of a difficult birth. Fortunately these kids often die soon after birth. They are probably best delivered by caesarean section.

Caesarean Section

Some difficult births are impossible to correct without resort to a caesarean operation (*see* plates 7.13–7.16). If a caesarean is performed the doe is often less damaged than if the delivery is made via the birth canal. Often the chance of kids surviving is increased as well. Your veterinary surgeon will obviously decide when and how it should be carried out. The approach is through the left-hand flank and the operation carried out under sedation and local anaesthesia. Alternatively a general anaesthetic may

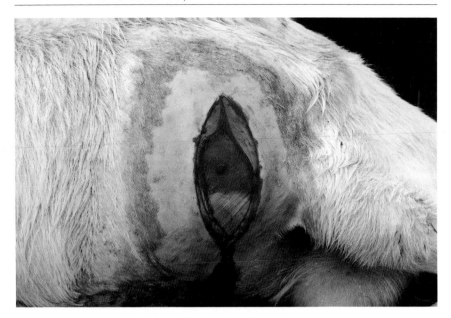

PLATE 7.13 Opening the left flank for a Caesarian section

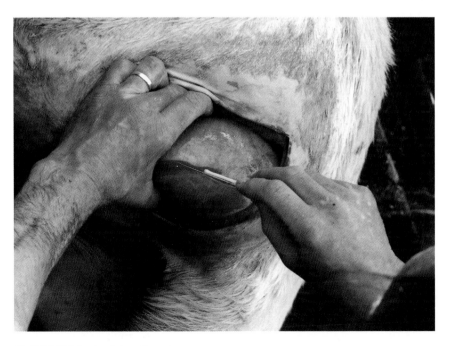

PLATE 7.14 Incising the uterus

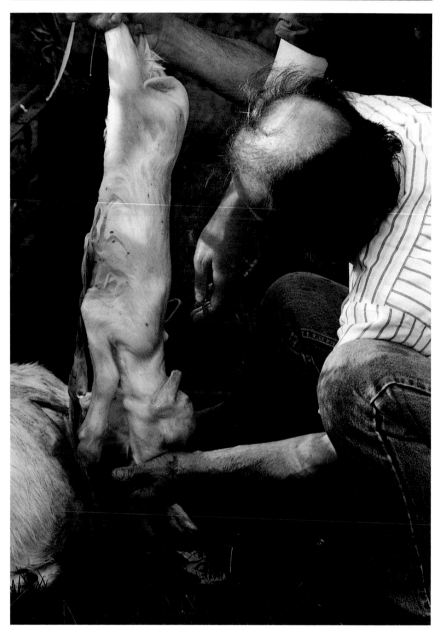

PLATE 7.15   Removing the kid which was too large for the small mother
to deliver naturally

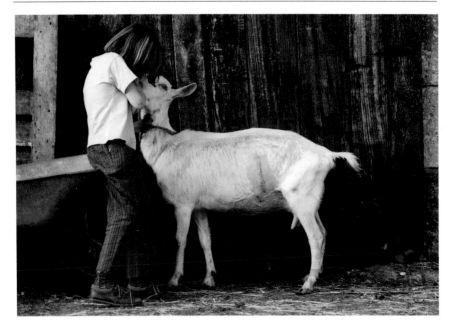

PLATE 7.16   The wound one week after the Caesarian section

be given (ketamine–xylazine mixture). Of course, if general anaesthesia is used then the doe must be intubated.

REVIVING KIDS

A protracted kidding gives rise to a sequel of events that are detrimental to the kid's survival. Firstly, the mother's contractions reduce the placental oxygenation, which makes the survival chances poorer for the kid. Secondly, the resistance in the kid's lung circulation is increased, making it more difficult for it to breathe. Complex biochemical changes occur, leading to acidosis in the kid. Thus after a difficult kidding or caesarean section, your vet may give the newborn kid a respiratory stimulant (such as 'Dopram-V'), and even injections of glucose and sodium bicarbonate. The glucose quickly supplies energy to the brain and nervous tissue, and the sodium bicarbonate is to counteract the acidosis.

Kidding is a very dangerous time for the kid, and attention to revival, and providing warmth cannot be overemphasised.

After the Kidding

Ensure that doe and kids are comfortable and leave them alone as much as possible. If possible leave the doe alone with her kids, not with other goats or the kids will become confused. Dress the navels of the kids with a suitable antiseptic such as tincture of iodine. From a discreet distance, try to observe if the kids drink colostrum. If they do not suck within six hours assist them to do so. Feel each kid's stomach to assess if it has sucked or not. The unfed kid feels empty whereas the abdomen of the full kid feels more like a ball. (*See* 'Feeling the kid's stomach for fullness' page 26.)

Prolapse of the Uterus

Very occasionally, the doe will continue to strain after kidding and push out her uterus. You will see a large red ball of tissue protruding from the vulva, which may be bleeding (*see* Plate 7.17).

This is an **emergency** and the first thing to do is to call your veterinary surgeon. Do not attempt to do anything because chasing the doe around will probably result in this delicate organ being bruised and possibly torn. Whilst awaiting the vet, organise some buckets of hot and cold water, for washing purposes.

Treatment
Eversion of the uterus may result in bleeding, shock and infection. After cleaning the uterus, your veterinary surgeon will quickly attempt to replace it and secure it into position again.

He may give the doe an epidural anaesthetic, in an attempt to stop her straining, or he may simply raise the back legs of the doe in order to eliminate the straining. He will control infection by placing pessaries (or tablets) directly into the uterus. The vulva is normally sutured or clipped to avoid a recurrence of the prolapse (*see* Plates 7.18 and 7.19).

After-care
Providing the uterus is replaced within a few hours the doe should survive. The owner must be observant to make sure that the doe does not start straining again when the vet has left. There may be sutures or retaining clips to be removed from the doe after about five days.

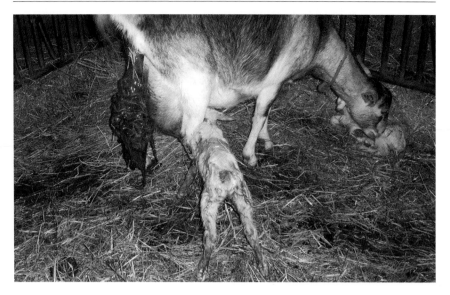

PLATE 7.17 Prolapsed uterus

Retained Placenta (Afterbirth)

Normally the afterbirth is pushed out from the uterus, within three hours of the birth. Should the doe fail to cleanse herself within fourteen hours, then contact your veterinary surgeon. Do not just pull the afterbirth or it may break, leaving part of it in the uterus.

Treatment normally involves antibiotics to control possible infections. These may be in the form of pessaries ('tablets' inserted into the uterus) or by injection. If the doe is very depressed and running a high temperature (greater then 39.5°C) seek advice from your vet more urgently (*see* plate 7.20).

Overdue Kidding

If a doe goes over 154 days of pregnancy (count the day of service as day zero), it may be advisable to have her checked by your veterinary surgeon. There may be something preventing her having the kids, for example, a mild hypocalcaemia. The longer

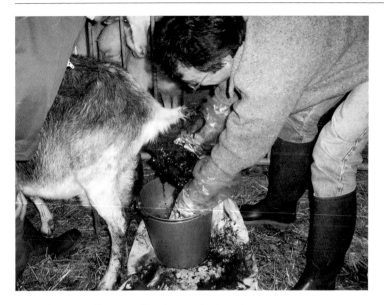

PLATE 7.18   Preparation for replacing the uterus.

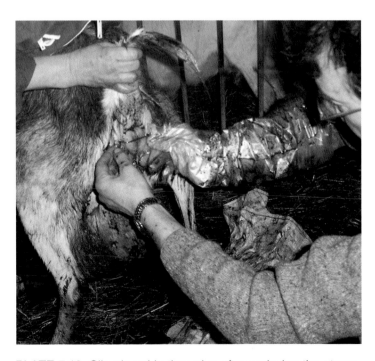

PLATE 7.19 Clip placed in the vulva after replacing the uterus.

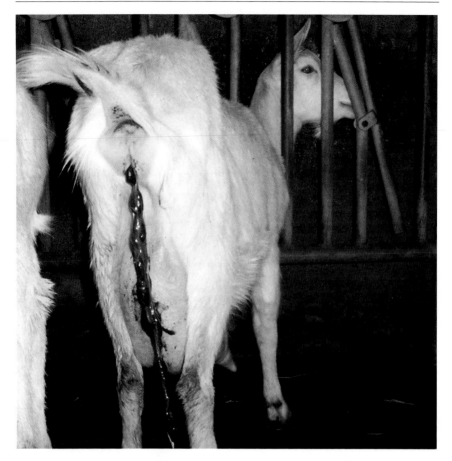

PLATE 7.20   Retained placenta

she goes on, the larger the kids grow. Large kids can present problems at birth and your vet may decide to induce the birth by injecting the doe with prostaglandin or a corticosteroid drug.

HOW MANY KIDS TO EXPECT

One study of Saanen goats in the United Kingdom revealed that one kid is common in the first pregnancy, but the average is 1.4 kids. Does that had kidded previously gave birth to an average of 2 kids. The distribution is:

	% of pregnancies
1 kid	20%
2 kids	60%
3 kids	18%
4 kids	2%
	100%

Very occasionally quintuplets are produced (*see* plate 7.21).

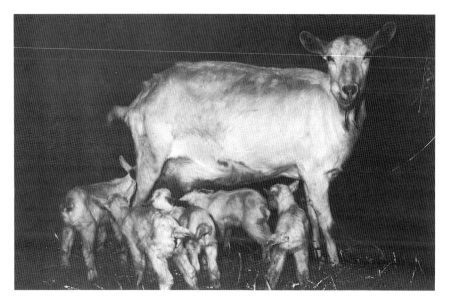

PLATE 7.21   Quintuplets born at the NIRD

METRITIS

After the kidding, the womb occasionally becomes infected and this is described as metritis. It may follow a retained placenta, a difficult kidding or just occur after a normal birth. Some discharge of mucus, often blood-tinged, is quite normal 2–3 days after kidding.

Symptoms
A discharge with colour ranging from dark brown through yellow can be seen coming from the doe's vulva. The goat may be quite sick and go off her food. It will be necessary to call your

veterinary surgeon who may treat the condition in any number of ways. He may decide to put tablets into the uterus, if the neck of the womb has not closed, or he may decide to irrigate the uterus using a catheter. If the cervix has closed, injections of antibiotics are generally successful.

MUMMIFIED KIDS

Occasionally a mummified kid will be produced. Mummification occurs after a kid has died in the womb, as a result of an infection, for example. Sometimes they are born as at the same time as a live twin (as in the plate below).

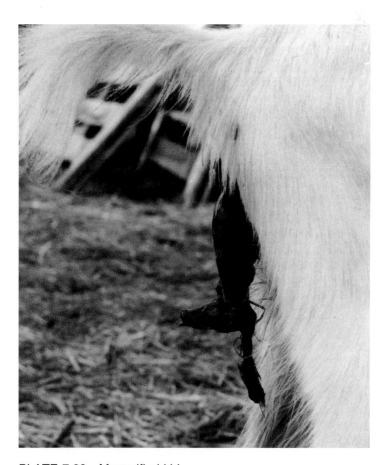

PLATE 7.22   Mummified kid

Embryo Transfer (ET)

This technique has been much in the news over the last three decades. Its application to the breeding of fibre goats (Angora) has been widespread.

The commercial value of Angora goats has meant that it is financially of greatest advantage to the owner of such a goat to produce as many progeny as possible in its lifetime. This is achieved in the case of a doe by using other less valuable females to carry fertilised eggs for her, in order to produce more (Angora) kids quickly.

The Technique
1. The donor's reproductive cycle is carefully observed.
2. The donor is super-ovulated, i.e. injected with hormones such as PMSG (pregnant mare serum gonadotropin) to obtain more eggs per ovulation than would normally occur.
3. She is mated to a selected sire so that many eggs, perhaps 9 to 12, become fertilised.
4. Commercially less valuable recipient does are organised by using prostaglandins to get them cycling in exact unison with the donor.
5. Approximately 4 days after the mating the fertilised eggs are surgically removed from the donor. This may involve a general anaesthetic and sophisticated equipment.
6. The eggs are placed into the wombs of the recipients using a pipette via a small surgical flank incision.

Refinements to the technique are continually being developed, reducing the procedure to minimise the interference to the goat.

The recipients are allowed to carry the embryo to full term. The kids born to the recipient are genetically unrelated to the foster mother. Thus perhaps 10 kids could be produced in the same 5 months from the same Angora. In theory she could be operated on frequently during one season.

One has to think carefully of the ethical considerations of such a technique, i.e. is it humane to subject the donor to such an operation. In my view it is questionable but the development of non-surgical techniques may eventually improve the situation.

A SUMMARY OF THE GOATKEEPER'S BREEDING YEAR

This guide is general and not applicable to all herds. It depends upon the individual herd history.

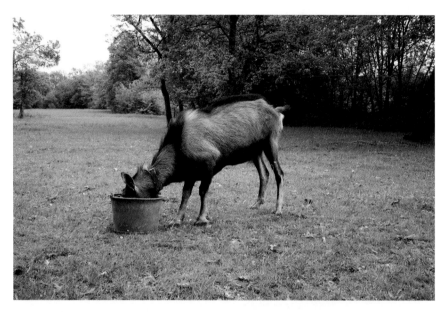

PLATE 7.23   Increase the buck's ration before the breeding season

BEFORE MATING

1. Vaccination:
   - Chlamydiosis vaccine for herds having had abortion problems in preceding season. Single injection to be carried out 1 month before service. Only young stock.
   - Footrot vaccine (if required).
   - Clostridial vaccine.

2. Possibly worming (depends on herd programme).
3. Prepare bucks for mating by feeding adequate ration. Especially important when sponging for early mating.
4. Sponging for females (if practised) to advance the season.
5. Worm the farm dogs.
6. Decide on cull goats – examine production records, look at condition of teeth before mating.

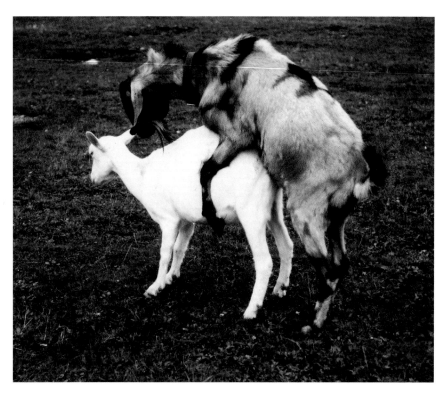

PLATE 7.24   Normal mating

DURING PREGNANCY

Early Pregnancy
1. Avoid all unnecessary handling and treatment during the first month of pregnancy.

2. Consider pregnancy checks.
   - Milk Test
   - Scan
3. Have abortions checked, especially if more than 3% of the herd.

Mid-pregnancy

1. Drying off. Herd therapy with antibiotics (if routine); otherwise treatment with dry cow infusions of any does with a history of mastitis.
2. Antiparasitic treatments. Once the goats are dry, various wormers with a long milk withdrawal time may be used. Invermectin may also be used at this stage for the treatment of Oestrus ovis larvae.
3. Vaccinations.
   - Orf, 4 to 6 weeks before the kidding date
   - Pasteurellosis (if necessary)
4. Milking machine function check. Consult a technically competent person to check pulsations, vacuum levels, etc.
5. Have abortions checked, especially if more than 3% of the herd.

Late Pregnancy

1. Gradually increase the concentrate ration.
2. Make preparations for kiddings: pens, etc.
3. Kidding box kits
4. Vaccination for clostridial diseases (enterotoxaemia/tetnus, etc) during the last two weeks of pregnancy. Check vaccine packet, as not all are licensed for use in pregnancy. Vaccination in early pregnancy may cause abortion. It is probably best to avoid clostridial vaccination altogether during pregnancy.

BIRTH (KIDDING)

1. Dress navels, e.g. tincture of iodine.
2. Separate mother and kid from other goats for 24 hours.
3. Afterbirth-note whether delivered or not.
4. Identify the kid.

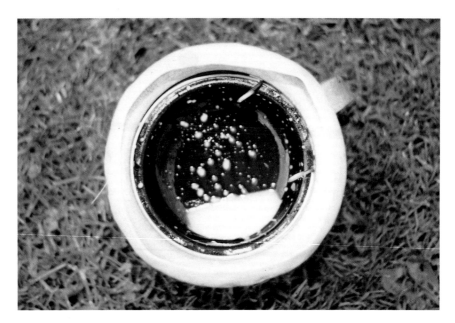

PLATE 7.25   Check the milking machine carefully to avoid mastitis in the next lactation

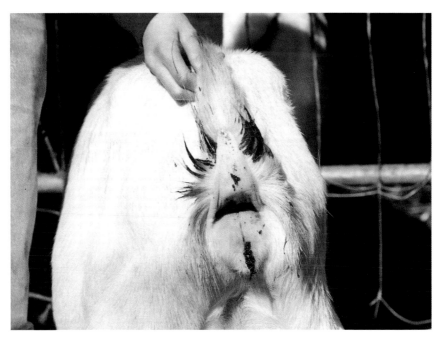

PLATE 7.26   Normal post-kidding 'gritty' discharge: no cause for alarm

KIDS AND GOATLINGS

(N.B. Not applicable to every farm)

1. Check female kids for two normal teats.
2. Check for umbilical hernias (large lump around navel in day-old kid).
3. Keep your eye on navels for sighs of navel ill.
4. Disbud breeding stock kids at about 4 days.
5. Johne's disease vaccine first 2 to 3 weeks after birth (if necessary).
6. Enterotoxaemia vaccine 8-in-1 type.
   - Kids from unvaccinated mothers at two weeks of age.
   - Kids born to vaccinated mothers at 12 weeks and 16 weeks.
7. Pasteurellosis vaccine (if necessary).
8. Worm treatments if at pasture.
9. Vaccination against chlamydia (if necessary).
10. Monitor the coccidiosis situation.

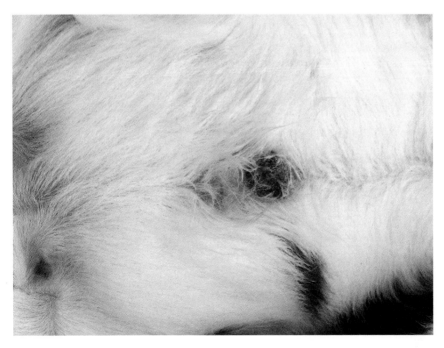

PLATE 7.27   Remember to treat navels in order to prevent infections as on this kid.

Chapter 8

OTHER CONDITIONS

GENERAL

ABSCESSES

Frequently found on goats, abscesses are local pockets of infection which contain pus. They tend to arise following small cuts which penetrate the skin. Germs entering at the same time as the cuts are responsible for the infection, and bacteria frequently isolated from abscesses include corynebacteria, staphylococci and streptococci.

Symptoms
Swelling will be found below the skin anywhere on the goat's body. The problem is that blood-blisters, growths, cysts and other conditions all look and feel rather similar to the layman.

Treatment
First of all do nothing, wait and see if the suspected abscess bursts. Bathing it in warm salt water may assist the pointing process. If nothing happens over a period of several days get your veterinary surgeon to examine it. Never incise a lump unless you are absolutely sure what it is.

Your vet will check what the lump is, and incise it if necessary. He may give the goat an injection of antibiotic depending upon the severity of the condition.

CASEOUS LYMPHADENITIS (C.L.A.)
(PSEUDOTUBERCULOSIS, ABSCESSES)

In the first edition of this book, I was able to write 'this condition does not occur in the UK'; unfortunately this is no longer the

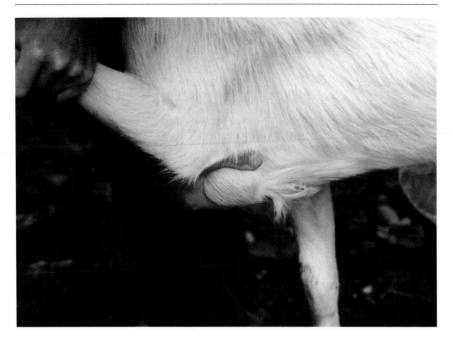

PLATE 8.1   Abscess on brisket (resulting from vaccination)

case. This infectious and contagious disease arrived in the UK with imported animals. The causal bacterium, *Corynebacterium pseudotuberculosis*, is a worldwide problem and it affects both sheep and goats. In countries such as France and the USA, the prevalence of the disease is high: in some infected herds half of the goats may have abscesses in their lymph nodes. The front part of the body is mainly affected, so the most commonly seen swelling is under the chin (the submandibular lymph node). The disease is chronic – a nuisance rather than a catastrophe. It causes work for the goatkeeper, some loss of herd performance and of course, unsightly goats.

Diagnosis
A smear or culture from the lymph node or abscess yields *C. pseudotuberculosis*. In countries where the disease is widespread, diagnosis is often by clinical inspection, the swellings being in constant sites, always following the lymphatic system.

Treatment
Carefully incise the abscess and drain out the pus. Your vet will

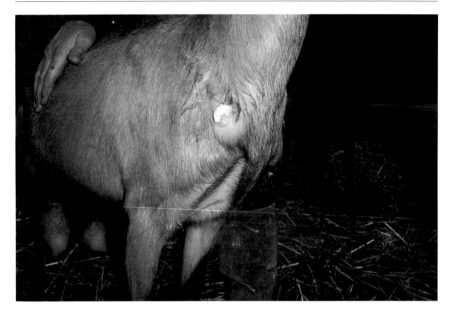

PLATE 8.2   Goat with caseous lymphadenitis abscess

guide you on the whole procedure and how to irrigate the abscess cavity after draining it.

Spread
The agent can be spread from the discharging abscess on an infected goat to other goats directly, or to the surroundings and hence to other goats. Infection can be by mouth, or through small cuts and abrasions in the skin. The bacterium then lodges in the lymph node draining that region of the body and multiplies there, causing a swelling. Experimentally it takes about 95 days from infection to the formation of abscesses.

If you are unfortunate enough to have this problem in your herd it is important not to allow the abscesses to burst and contaminate the environment. It is much better to incise and drain them in a careful manner and dispose of all the contents and swabs etc by incineration. Try and choose the time when the abscess is ready to burst. This will probably result in a better 'clear-up' than incising too early on in the abscess formation. The organism can survive in the goathouse for long periods and possibly infect other goats.

Control

- Run a closed herd.
- Quarantine incoming goats for long periods (three months or more if possible).
- Take care when introducing goats with unusual swellings into your herd.
- Avoid contact at shows and sales.
- Avoid all physical causes of injury that help to allow infection of the skin – sharp corners, splintered wood etc.
- Avoid wooden 'furniture' in goat houses as it is harder to disinfect than metal.
- Remember transmission can occur through instruments, tattoo equipment, ear tags etc.
- Vaccines. No vaccine of proven efficacy has yet been developed (although there are vaccines on the market). No licensed vaccine is available in the UK as yet but researchers are optimistic that they will be available within the next few years.

Note: Many different germs can be involved with abscess formation, but this disease is a specific type of infection.

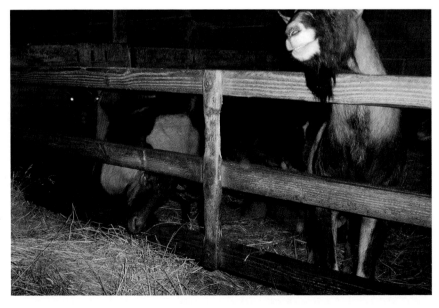

PLATE 8.3   Avoid wooden furniture in the goathouse

ANTHRAX

Anthrax, which is a notifiable disease, is an acute fever produced by a germ *Bacillus anthracis* and generally resulting in sudden death of the animal. The same bacterium can cause disease in other animals such as cattle, sheep, pigs and even humans.

Symptoms
Animals are found dead or very sick with a temperature well above normal, for instance, 41°C (106°F).

Occurrence
This is very, very rare, in the United Kingdom because of the regulations imposed by Defra. Over the years this control has reduced the prevalence to an extremely low level in all species. All stock-owners are obliged to report sudden deaths (cases where the owners see no signs of sickness prior to the death). These deaths are investigated by Defra staff, who check the dead animals' blood for the presence of anthrax bacteria. Positive cases are incinerated on site, without being cut open. This is because the organism forms spores when in contact with the air. Spores are long-lived and can inhabit the soil for fifty years. Thus if the carcase is incinerated unopened the chance of future disease is eliminated. Anthrax is a worldwide problem and is especially prevalent in the western United States. In most countries it is a 'reportable disease' meaning suspected cases must be notified to the government veterinary service.

Treatment and Control
Animals are rarely treated because death is so rapid. In the UK, should goatkeepers be suspicious, they are obliged to contact either Defra (Animal Health Division) or their veterinary surgeon. There is no charge for this.

'In contact' goats would be treated with large doses of intramuscular penicillin. The clean up and disinfection of the affected premises would be supervised by the State Veterinary Service (SVS).

Vaccines to control anthrax are used in many countries but they are under the control of the government veterinary service of each country. They are not available for use in the UK.

ARTHRITIS AND JOINT DISEASE

Septic Arthritis

Arthritis may follow any generalised infection or bacteraemia (blood poisoning). The organisms settle in the joints, causing degenerative change and pain. Success with such cases depends upon how quickly treatment is started, but the outlook is often bleak.

Symptoms
The goat is very lame and swellings may be detected at the joints. Because of the pain resulting from the swellings the goats tend to lie down most of the time.

Treatment
Antibiotic injections may be prescribed by your veterinary surgeon but the damage is often so great that the goat fails to get better.

Prevention
Because this condition frequently follows an infection of the navel, cleanliness at birth is important. Dressing the navel of kids with tincture of iodine should prevent this type of infection.

Arthritis Associated with Mycoplasma

In Australia, Continental Europe and the USA caprine *M. mycoides var. mycoides* (large colony type) has been associated with a variety of syndromes including arthritis. *M. capricolium* causes a septicaemia followed by pneumonia and arthritis in goats. (This infection is not present in the UK.)

Diagnosis relies upon laboratory examination and culture of the germ from the joints. Certain antibiotics can be used for treatment, which may involve the whole herd.

Non-septic Arthritis

This is a temporary problem resulting from an increased quantity of fluid in the joints.

Symptoms
Swelling of the joints, probably following twisting or sprain. The affected joint is swollen and painful but the goat is bright and continues to eat.

Treatment
Essentially rest, possibly supporting the joint with an elastic bandage to reduce further movement. With time the excess fluid is re-absorbed and the lameness disappears.

Caprine Arthritis Encephalitis Virus (Big Knee, CAE)

This viral disease is encountered in North America and Europe including the UK. In France the disease is present in 80 to 90 per cent of herds, but is much less prevalent in the British Isles. The virus is a retrovirus (lentivirus) and has a long incubation period of up to several years. It is extremely similar to but distinct from maedi-visna in sheep. Virologists argue as to whether or not it is a different virus. In the UK, after the disease was recognised, many goatkeepers carried out blood tests on their herds, eliminated reactors and the spread of the disease was fairly limited. Some countries have introduced schemes to try and reduce prevalence. This usually means creating two sub-herds and milking them separately. Goatkeepers must remain ever diligent, however, because symptomless carriers may introduce the virus into clean herds.

Symptoms
Arthritis affecting many joints is the predominant feature of CAE (caprine arthritis encephalitis) virus infection in mature goats. Usually the front legs are involved, the carpii (knees) being the most frequently affected joint. Often both sides are swollen at the same time. The other joints, hocks, stifles, fetlocks and hips may be involved.

Symptoms can range from mild to severe, from slight swelling of the knees to sudden severe lameness, in which case the animal should be put down on humane grounds. Characteristically, the joint swelling is often noted before the symptoms of lameness become apparent. The reduced milk production is estimated to be 100 kg in a first lactation. Sometimes the udder is affected becoming hard and unproductive with often just one half being affected. The encephalitis part of the disease affects growing kids aged from 1–5 months, causing nervous signs. The kids become unable to stand, the head is twisted to one side, and when down they may show paddling symptoms with their forelegs.

The disease process
The virus tends to lodge in the bone marrow and is reactivated by stress. The strain of the kidding and lactation is probably the

main cause in dairy goats. Often many animals in a herd may be infected, even before any disease symptoms are noted. The virus is most unpredictable in its disease-causing ability. French workers estimate that seventy per cent of infected animals show no symptoms.

Spread of the disease

As with HIV-Aids in humans, it would seem that infected cells have to be transferred between goats in order to pass on the virus. The most likely time of infection is probably around kidding, when transmission occurs from the doe to the kids in the colostrum and nasal secretions. Milk and colostrum are thought to be the primary methods of spread.

Casual contact is unlikely to result in the infection being passed on. Infection of kids in the uterus is thought to be rare. There is no evidence of transmission by semen from infected male goats to the females. It is theoretically possible to transmit the disease by needles from one goat to the next.

Control

There is no treatment for this condition. Periodic blood testing of goats should be followed by the culling of any reacting to the agar gel immuno-diffusion test (AGIDT). The ELISA test is also useful in detecting infected animals earlier than the AGIDT. It is at present more expensive. If a herd is known to be infected then kids should be removed from the doe immediately after kidding, before she can lick them; the aim is to prevent infection being passed on. The colostrum is then milked from the udder and 'thermalised', i.e. heated up to 56°C for one hour to destroy any virus. When at a suitable temperature the colostrum is fed to the kid. From then on the kid is fed on artificial milk.

Blood testing goats in late pregnancy enables the owner to identify reactors before the kidding, so that special attention can be given to them at the birth. No successful vaccine has yet been developed but the French are carrying out trials with such vaccines, in their goats.

Post mortem findings

A proliferative synovitis and a periarthritis can be noted in affected joints.

AUJESZKY'S DISEASE (PSEUDORABIES)

Aujeszky's disease is a viral disease affecting primarily the pig, but occasionally causing disease in goats kept in close contact with pigs. When it does affect goats, it can be a very serious problem. Aujeszky's disease has a wide geographical distribution. It is present in Europe, North and South America, North Africa and Asia.

Symptoms
Unlike the situation in cattle, where the disease is also called the 'mad itch', no evidence of skin irritation is seen. The goats quickly develop symptoms of restlessness, sweating, screaming and finally paralysis. The course of the disease can be fairly rapid; some goats dying within twenty-four hours. In one outbreak in Holland, thirteen out of fifteen died in a space of ten days. Diagnosis can be made from either blood samples or microscopic examination of the brain.

Control
The disease is absent in the United Kingdom, even in pigs. In other parts of the world, if a premises is known to have the disease in the pig herd it would be sensible to keep the goats away from the pigs. As the disease is eradicated from the pig population the potential problem will disappear for goatkeepers.

BORDER DISEASE

I shall mention this problem for completeness although the disease is rarely diagnosed in goats. In sheep a disease causing a mixture of different symptoms, abortion and nervous signs is caused by this pestivirus. It is probably present in most of the world. In New Zealand the lambs are called 'hairy shakers'. In goats the symptoms are extremely ill-defined. Stress is known to play an important part in the disease process.

CANCERS IN GOATS (TUMOURS, NEOPLASIA)

A cancer is the accumulation of tissue which results when cells suddenly start to multiply at a rate above normal. The reasons why they commence to multiply out of hand like this are largely unknown. We know that some of them are associated with viruses, but cancer as yet is still the subject of much research. Probably the most comforting fact for goatkeepers to hear is that the frequency of cancers in goats is not particularly high.

The results of the two following studies puts the problem into perspective. Only fifteen out of 2,500 goats were affected in one United States survey and only seventy out of 800,000 in another abattoir survey. A second piece of information to remove concern from goatkeepers is that no one particular type of cancer seems to be a problem.

Conjunctivitis (Pink Eye), Contagious Ophthalmia

This is a fairly common problem in goatherds. The symptoms are a reddening of the white of the eye and generally a pussy discharge. The causal agent can be one of several different types of micro-organism including mycoplasma, rickettsia and bacteria. The bacteria are often secondary invaders which make the problem worse. The problem occurs in most countries.

Many factors may be involved in predisposing to the disease and these include dust and overcrowding of goats.

The eye must be carefully examined to ensure that a foreign body is not the cause; grass seeds commonly get into the eyes of goats. Normally several goats are involved when conjunctivitis occurs and it may affect only one or both eyes.

Remember that similar signs may accompany viral respiratory infections of the goat when coughing etc. is noticed, i.e. a viral conjunctivitis. In these cases the cause is the respiratory virus itself.

Treatment
Generally the condition responds quickly to eye ointments containing antibiotics such as chloramphenicol and cloxacillin.

Cystitis

From time to time does develop an infection of the bladder; it is possibly more common in animals that have had assisted deliveries. The symptoms include frequent urination, when only a small amount of urine is passed. There may be blood and or pus in the

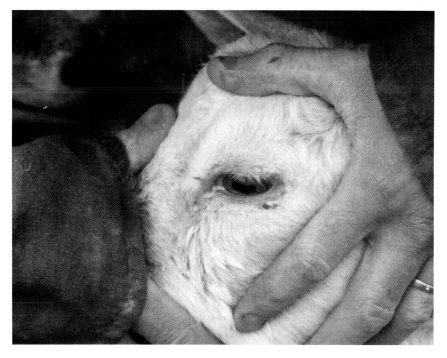

PLATE 8.4   Conjunctivitis

urine and often the perineal skin is wet with urine. Sometimes reduced milk yield, dullness and signs of discomfort (teeth grinding) may be noticed.

Treatment
Antibiotic injections will normally restore the goat to full health. Cystitis in males is not common except when associated with urinary calculi. Readers will be aware of the frequent urination pattern of the buck in the breeding season. This should not be confused with cystitis.

FOOT-AND-MOUTH DISEASE

This highly contagious viral disease of all cloven-hoofed animals is not normally present in the United Kingdom.

It has been eradicated from much of the world: Europe (the

EU), Australia, New Zealand and North America. High speed transport and the highly contagious nature of the disease means that it always presents a potential threat to any country. In the EU, as with many countries it is controlled by slaughter of the affected animals, compensation being paid by the government. Because it spreads so rapidly, all owners must report suspicious symptoms immediately; I describe them below. If you suspect foot-and-mouth disease phone either your veterinary surgeon, or the government veterinary service. Do not delay; there will be no charge made to you, even in the event of a false alarm.

Symptoms
Blisters or 'vesicles' form in any of the following places: lips, tongue, dental pad, teats, or the coronary band of the hoof. Affected animals tend to become lame and possibly salivate excessively. It is normally very mild, almost unapparent in the goat.

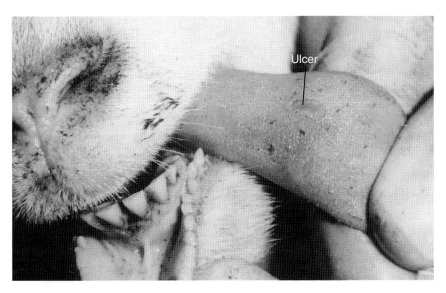

PLATE 8.5   Foot-and-mouth disease – tongue ulcer

Control
Many countries, including the European Union, have a slaughter policy and treatment is never considered. The State Veterinary Service will deal with all aspects of the outbreak if it is confirmed.

Legal aspects of foot-and-mouth disease
This is a *notifiable disease* and owners are legally obliged to report any suspicious cases as soon as possible.

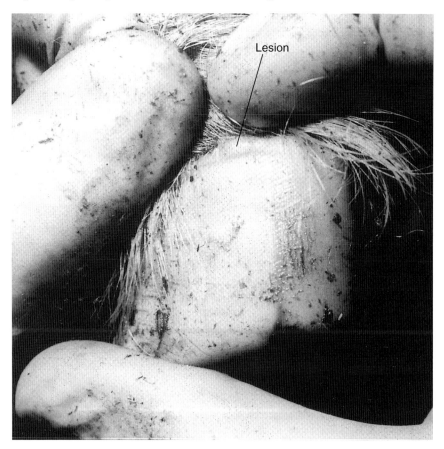

PLATE 8.6   Foot-and-mouth disease – lesion on the coronary band

LEPTOSPIROSIS

There are few reported cases of this bacterial disease, that results from infection with leptospiral organisms. It can result in either a very acute disease following blood poisoning, or a mild form may be seen. In contrast to cattle the abortion form is not characteristic of goats, except as a complication of blood poisoning. A survey of goats in Morocco revealed that over a quarter of them had antibodies to the organism, suggesting that infection may be quite common. It is probably the case that sub-clinical lepto-spirosis is fairly widespread. In France, an examination of sera from 363 goats suspected of having leptospirosis revealed only 2.5 per cent positive ones. The serotypes most frequently found were icterohaemorrhagica, grippotyphosa and canicola. It has not been recorded on the UK VIDA system.

Spread of the disease
It is more common in warm, humid climates on alkaline soils and with surface water.

The organism is generally spread from one animal to another by urine, which often contaminates water supplies. The infection tends to settle in the kidney and thereby infects the urine. After infection, goats are known to harbour the bacterium in their kidneys for at least a month.

Symptoms
Most animals are found dead. Some show dullness and specific symptoms, occasionally with jaundice. Sometimes, after the blood-poisoning phase the bacterium may remain in the nervous system and produce symptoms of encephalitis (inflammation of the brain).

Treatment
In many cases discovery is too late for treatment but it may be beneficial to try and prevent carrier animals spreading the disease. Your veterinary surgeon will advise you on these aspects.

Note: Zoonose. Some forms of leptospirosis are transmissible to humans.

LISTERIOSIS (CIRCLING DISEASE)

Listeriosis is the disease caused by the bacterium *Listeria monocytogenes*. In goats it shows up in three forms; one affecting the brain, causing circling symptoms, the second being respon-sible for some cases of abortion. The third type is septicaemia or blood poisoning. It is not very common; for example, the VLA[*] laboratories only diagnose the problem in two or three samples

[*] Veterinary Laboratory Agency, an agent of Defra.

each year. There are other members of the listeria family but these are not disease causing.

Symptoms
Symptoms of the circling form are initially dullness, possibly with the goat head-pressing against an object. In my experience the first symptom is that of a lowered (dropped) ear on the affected side. Later the animal tends to turn its head to one side and progresses to walk in circles. Often brown rumen contents are seen at the lips. Over the period of a week, the affected goat becomes progressively weaker until it goes down, unable to rise. There may be a rise in temperature to about 42°C. Your veterinary surgeon will have to examine the goat in order to differentiate this disease from several others. Many goats die within four days.

Abortions due to *Listeria* may reach 15 per cent of an affected group. They are reported to occur from three months of pregnancy onwards.

Spread of the disease
The organism is present in the soil, and it must be stressed, is quite widespread. It may be present in faeces and silages. Infection can occur through the conjunctiva of the eye or from taking the organism in by mouth. There are thought to be special predisposing reasons why infection occurs and one of them is feeding silage and haylage. The reason for this is that the organism thrives in poorly made silage (pH>4.2) especially if it is badly contaminated with soil. It is perhaps fortunate that few goatkeepers feed silage in the United Kingdom. However, soil may contaminate other foods if goats are badly managed and allowed to jump into hayracks and feeders. The practice of feeding maize silage to goats is increasing in many countries, bringing with it the increased prevalence of listeriosis. One North American study found a higher risk of the disease in browse-fed angora goats, compared to pasture and hay fed animals.

Treatment
Poor response is obtained if animals have developed the circling form of the disease but antibiotics such as penicillin or chlortetracycline may be tried. Ampicillin is reported to be the most effective by the French. Treatment should continue for ten days, if the symptoms improve after forty-eight hours. Once symptoms

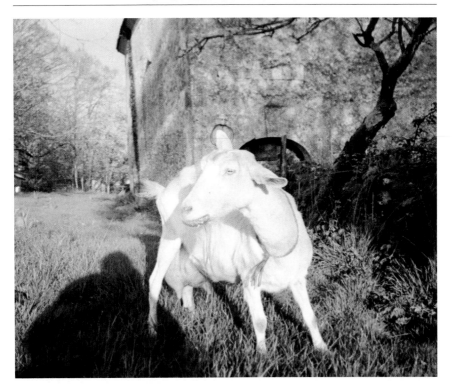

PLATES 8.7 & 8.8   Listeriosis in a goat

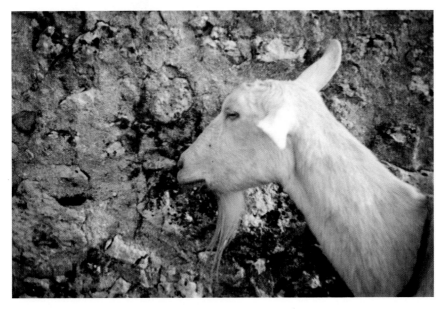

are noted in a herd, it would be sensible to check the in-contact animals for rises in body temperature. Fevered in-contact goats would probably benefit from preventive antibiotic treatment. In one outbreak, affecting fourteen adults and two kids, two adults and two kids died, the other adults responding to treatment with chlortetracycline. Treatment can often lead to disappointing results.

Prevention
Avoiding the spoilage of food by soil, especially if silage is fed, is important. Silage must be well made so as to ensure complete fermentation in order to prevent the organism multiplying in it. The mystery of why silage causes listeriosis when contaminated is still being studied. It seems that some factor in silage allows the bacterium to invade the goat. It is postulated that the silage in some way reduces the goat's defence mechanism.

Many researchers consider that immunodepression (a reduced ability of the immune system to respond to challenges) is why some animals succumb to the infection and not others. Keeping goats healthy and reducing other disease challenges will help to prevent listeriosis. Probiotics are reported to be of value when fed with the silage, even when risky silage is fed.

No vaccine of proven value is available.

Note: Listeriosis can affect humans and care must be taken when dealing with aborted kids and placentas.

Listeria and cheese production
Cheese can be contaminated by the listeria germ, and this is responsible for outbreaks of disease in humans. Listeria can multiply at low temperatures (down to 0°C). It is killed by pasteurisation. Goat cheeses are normally made at acidities (pH) lower than 4.5. This is also a security, as the germ cannot survive a pH lower than 5.0.

MAEDI-VISNA (MV)

This chronic pneumonia of sheep was recently diagnosed for the first time in the United Kingdom; maedi-visna can also infect goats.

Symptoms
This disease is caused by a virus but it has an extremely long incubation period of at least two years. The symptoms are described as 'progressive', very slowly becoming more apparent. Listlessness and loss of weight become obvious and the animal breathes more rapidly than normal. Goats showing nervous symptoms have also been reported.

Treatment and Control
There is no treatment for this condition and slaughter of affected goats is the only answer. Blood samples can be tested to identify affected animals. Your vet would advise you, if you were unlucky enough to have this problem in your herd.

SCRAPIE

This unusual disease occurs in sheep and extremely rarely in goats. It is caused by a minute agent (a prion) which is smaller than a virus and results in a fatal brain disease.

It is present in many countries but not Australia or New Zealand. It has only been very rarely identified in goats, on recent abattoir surveys in the UK. The agent can survive for up to three years in the environment.

Symptoms
Scrapie gives rise to symptoms of abnormal gait and itchiness and goats may show depression or progressive weight loss. Caprines typically scratch themselves with their horns or feet. When I have examined scrapie goats, the striking symptom was their tendency to fall down when chased. They may show a range of nervous symptoms such as trembling and inco-ordination. Because it has a long incubation period (sometimes years), single cases are likely rather than many animals being affected at the same time. Some goats are just found dead and the diagnosis is only made at post-mortem examination.

Treatment
Scrapie is incurable, there is no vaccine available to control this disease and affected animals should be slaughtered. Goats can become infected from infected sheep but recent investigations

suggest that scrapie can occur in goats that have not had contact with sheep.

Avoiding Scrapie
Transmission occurs mainly from an infected placenta and less importantly through bodily fluids such as saliva, blood etc. Preventing the eating of placentae and general kidding hygiene may help but culling clinical cases is important.

Diagnosis
The post-mortem diagnosis of scrapie is by laboratory examination or samples of brain tissue. Using an electron microscope, scrapie-associated fibrils may be seen. Scrapie is a T.S.E (a Transmissible Spongiform Encephalopathy) it is similar to BSE in cattle and CJD in humans. In many countries (including the EU) it is notifiable if suspected.

Action in the UK
In the UK all suspected cases of scrapie must be reported to your local Animal Health Office of the SVS (Defra).

Compulsory slaughter
If scrapie is confirmed in goats in any EU country, compulsory slaughter of the herd will follow.

BSE in goats
One case of Bovine Spongiform Encephalopathy (BSE) has recently been identified in the carcase of a French goat. It is likely that the source of the infection was infected feed.

TUBERCULOSIS

Goats can occasionally contract tuberculosis (*Mycobacterium tuberculosis*). They can be infected with the human strain or *M.bovis* or *M.avium*.

The source of infection used to be mainly from tuberculous cattle. As the prevalence of TB in cattle is now low, infection in goats is almost unknown in the United Kingdom and the other developed countries. Cattle are tested in order to prevent tuberculous milk being consumed by humans, and goats running with cattle should be tested at the same time. Reservoirs of TB are thought to occur in species of wildlife which contaminate the pasture and this is another possible source of infection to goats. Goats are generally infected with the avian strain of TB but, very occasionally, the bovine strain has been recorded. Goatkeepers should seek guidance from their Veterinarian or State Veterinary Service as to the need to test their goats for TB. The test is carried out by injecting tuberculin into the skin and checking the reaction after 72 hours. Monitoring carcases at abattoirs is also a useful way of checking for the presence of this disease.

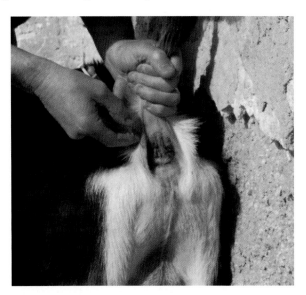

PLATE 8.9 TB test using the caudal fold

Symptoms
Generally weight loss and sometimes respiratory signs.

Control
Goats reacting to the skin test would be culled.

URINARY CALCULI (STONES IN THE BLADDER)

Male goats are especially prone to blockage of the urethra by 'stones' which collect in the bladder. If the stones leave the bladder and pass into the narrow penis, they cause obstruction and blockage to urine flow.

Symptoms
The goat rapidly becomes distressed and repeatedly attempts to urinate; crystals may be noticed on the belly hair. Place the goat on a dry concrete surface and observe to see if he can pass any urine. Sometimes the pressure becomes so great that the bladder bursts and urine floods into the abdominal cavity. This may result in the goat becoming brighter for a few days because the pain associated with the blockage disappears.

Treatment
Sometimes the obstruction can be relieved by surgery; I find only about half of the cases are successful. The operation would not normally be performed on a breeding male because it may affect his fertility.

Prevention
The main predisposing cause of this condition is dirty drinking water buckets. Goats will not drink dirty water and if their water is not clean they will ration themselves. Stall-fed males on a high concentrate/low roughage diet are particularly at risk. Decreasing the concentrate may help to avoid the problem. It may also be prudent to avoid concentrates that are high in calcium.

Plate 8.10 illustrates the type of stones (or calculi) found in the bladder of a goat that was suffering from this problem.

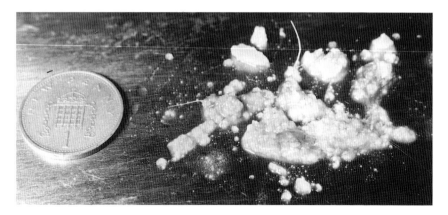

PLATE 8.10   Calculi from the bladder of a goat suffering from urinary obstruction

TRANSIT TETANY

Sometimes goats undergoing a journey become weak and go down, unable to rise. The condition can normally be reversed by the injection of calcium and magnesium solutions.

SKIN DISEASES

Some diseases causing damage to the skin have been described in other chapters. (See ORF, page 130, and also pages 127–129 and 137.)

DERMATOPHILOSIS (*Cutaneous streptotrichosis*)

This is a chronic skin disease of humid climates recently reported in goats in Italy. The bacterium *Dermatophilus congolensis* can be transmitted by contact with infected animals or by ectoparasites. The symptoms start with reddening of the skin followed by the production of greases or crusts. As it progresses the affected skin becomes scabby and crusty. In the Italian cases the disease commenced around ears and nose spreading to the head, neck and limbs. Treatment is difficult and the success influenced by climatic conditions. Antibiotics are generally used. It has not been recorded in the UK.

RINGWORM (DERMATOMYCOSES)

Despite the common name, this disease is a fungal condition and nothing to do with worms. Ringworm can affect all farm animals and it can be transmitted to humans. Normally a disease of the winter months, it is especially prevalent when animals are housed together. In goats several fungi can grow on the hair and skin; they include *Trichophyton verrucosum*.

Ringworm does relatively little harm to the goat, but it looks unsightly and it is a potential danger to humans.

Symptoms
A grey-white crusty appearance to small areas of skin should alert the goatkeeper to the possibility of ringworm infection. The

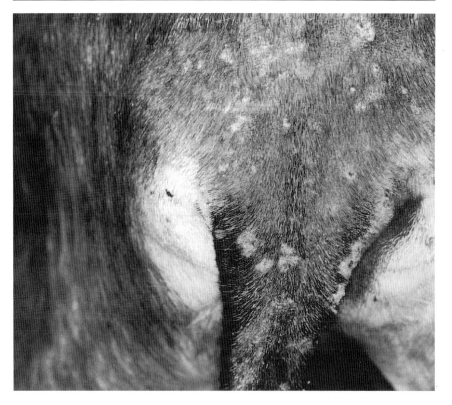

PLATE 8.11   Ringworm

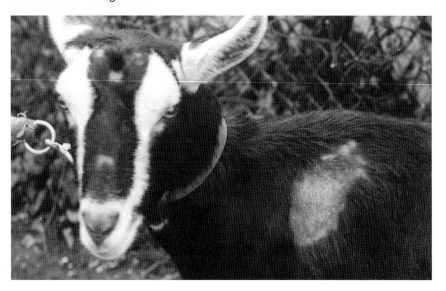

skin is usually thickened and the hairs thin or absent. There is generally no itching or evidence of irritation. Enlargement of the affected areas occurs over a period of weeks and different patches may join up to form one large area. The fungus in the middle tends to die, due to lack of oxygen and this accounts for the descriptive name, ringworm.

The Predisposing Causes
Warm, humid conditions are contributory to the growth of fungus on the hair and skin. Badly ventilated goathouses are ideal for its spread. Young animals tend to be more susceptible to ringworm than older animals. Spread of the disease is either by direct contact or from contact with contaminated objects.

Treatment
Recently Griseofulvin (oral) was withdrawn in the EU and only topical preparations are now available. For goats, one is obliged to use topical treatment with medicines licensed for other species such as Enilconazole (Janssen).

Prevention
The disease is best prevented by avoiding humid housing. Avoiding contact with contaminated objects, such as halters, can sometimes be difficult, even in the best-managed animals.

DISEASE CAUSED BY ECTOPARASITES

General comments on the control of external parasites in goats.

1. There are no products licensed for use on goats in the UK so vets are obliged to use products licensed for use in other species. Frequently these drugs are very toxic so read the information concerning operator safety and disposal of containers.

2. Residues can persist in the milk and meat of treated goats so take advice from your vet about withdrawal times for these, in order to prevent humans from ingesting toxic compounds. I have indicated some products licensed for use on goats in other countries, which may be helpful.

MANGES

Infestation of the skin by parasitic mites is referred to as mange. There are several types of mange which affect the goat; they are:

- Chorioptic mange
- Demodectic mange
- Psoroptic mange
- Sarcoptic mange

Although they are all caused by mites, it is important to know which one is affecting the goat. They are of varying significance, some causing only mild problems, others being virtually incurable. For this reason, your veterinary surgeon will probably take a sample for laboratory examination, in order to identify the mange involved.

Chorioptic Mange (Heel or Leg Mange)

The mites, *Chorioptes caprae*, infest the skin of the lower leg of goats. They are responsible for a little irritation and they cause the goat to look unsightly. Housed goats in the winter are more likely to suffer from the problem than grazing animals.

Symptoms and Treatment

Itchiness may be noticed and there may be small crusty scabs. It mainly affects the heel region.

Topical organophosphorous compounds are used in some countries, for example, chlorfenvinphos combined with alphamethrin (Bayer/Fort Dodge). This could be applied to the legs with a paint brush if only a few animals are affected. Be careful to cover all of the legs. A repeat treatment two weeks later would be advised. Ivermectin, by injection, is also very effective.

Demodectic Mange

The mites, *Demodex caprae*, invade the hair follicles and sebaceous glands of the skin. This causes a chronic inflammation and the development of small pustules or abscesses. The disease spreads slowly on the skin of affected goats. It does not spread rapidly from goat to goat. In France the problem is increasing, and it is thought that the keeping of goats in intensive conditions is conducive to the spread of the mange. Goatlings between the ages of 10 and 15 months are mainly affected.

Symptoms
Small lumps are noticed in the skin, varying in size from a match head up to a small pea. They may be like a cyst or bag of fluid. If incised the nodule can be squeezed and a thick waxy content forced out. Microscopic examination of the material will reveal the mite. Little irritation is noticed, probably because the mite is so deep-seated. The areas mostly affected are at the front of the animal: neck, shoulder and chest. The animals can become so severely affected that they eventually die.

Treatment
Response to treatment is generally poor. Drugs such as malathion are often ineffective, although success has been claimed recently for rotenone (Coopers Demodetic Mange Dressing). Some authors suggest cutting open the pustules and painting with tincture of iodine. You must discuss this problem with your veterinary surgeon.

Psoroptic Mange
This mite is found mainly in the ears of affected goats where it causes some irritation and head shaking. It may also extend to the poll and even to the legs. The variety of mite which causes sheep scab (*Psoroptes ovis*) is distinct from *Psoroptes communis caprae* which affects only goats.

Treatment.
Aerosol products containing permethrin are useful in that they can be directed down the ear canal. To kill subsequent stages that hatch from the eggs, a second treatment must be given to all the affected goats 10 to 14 days later. It would be wise to re-examine all the goats at regular intervals after treatment, to ensure that the problem has been fully controlled. The decision of whether to treat only the affected animals or the whole herd would need to be taken with your vet. An alternative and effective treatment is to give two injections of ivermectin with an interval of seven days.

Sarcoptic Mange
A serious mange causing crusty scabs on the skin is due to the mite *Sarcoptes scabei*. This form of mange appears to be more serious in goats than in other species of animals. The mites burrow in the skin and lay their eggs in tunnels. After hatching,

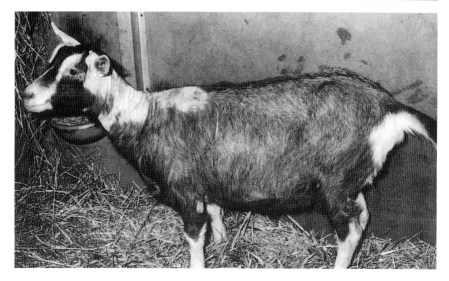

PLATE 8.12   Sarcoptic mange

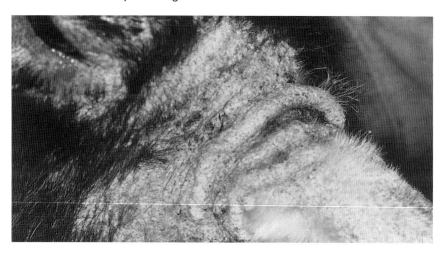

the nymphs work their way to the surface of the skin where they
become adults.

Symptoms
Scabby patches on the skin, especially on the head and neck,
causing itchiness, are characteristic of the disease. Affected
animals lose condition and appear very unsightly. Due to the

irritation caused by the mites the goats tend to rub and scratch and the affected areas get larger.

Treatment
Results are frequently disappointing. Goats often have to be destroyed after several months of unsuccessful treatment. Repeat washes with the acaricide (dip) have to be carried out because the eggs of the mite are not destroyed. Thus the repeat wash tends to kill the mites after they have hatched from the eggs.

There are reports of the use of ivermectin, by injection, to treat this condition. Two doses are given at a seven day interval. Although used in some countries, it is not licensed for use on goats in all countries. Permenthrin and piperonyl used together as a pour-on are licensed for non-lactating goats in the USA. The treatment should be repeated after two weeks.

Control
The microscopic mite can be spread from goat to goat either by direct contact or by equipment. Care should be taken to avoid using the same brushes, feeding pails and similar equipment for both infected and clean animals.

LICE INFESTATION

Lice are found in the coat and on the skin and are just visible to the naked eye.

There are two types of louse that affect goats; Biting lice which feed on the skin and scabs and sucking lice which have mouth-parts that pierce the skin to draw blood. Lice have a world-wide distribution but there are several different species and not all countries have the whole range. One fact about lice is that all the stages of development from eggs to adult take place on the goat. They cannot survive for very long off the goat. This is very important when considering methods of controlling them. The lice of cattle, sheep and goats are host specific and tend not to infest the other species.

Symptoms
Infestation with lice causes intense irritation and itching, they are especially noticeable in the winter months in Europe. Lice

populations tend to decrease in summer and increase in autumn and winter.

Goats with lice have dull, thin coats (*see* plate 8.14). They tend to be restless and groom themselves more than is normal. Transmission is mainly through direct contact between animals. In very severe cases heavy infestations of biting lice can cause anaemia.

Control
The goatkeeper has two choices: 1. To attempt to eradicate the lice and 2. To live with them but reduce the numbers periodically.

The ultimate aim of herd owners should be to eradicate this parasite from their animals. It is quite possible in a closed herd with adequate planning. Treatments effective against lice are applied twice, with an interval of two weeks. By this programme the (insecticide-resistant) eggs hatch 9 to 12 days after the first treatment and the second application kills the susceptible stages which develop from these newly hatched eggs. A suggested strategy for this is detailed below.

Eradication plan
Most of the life cycle of the lice takes place on the goat but since they are only able to survive for a few days off the host the goatkeeper needs to have a time when the goathouse is completely rested. Sometimes this is possible in dairy herds when the milkers dry off in late autumn.

Step one. Treat all the goats including, bucks and kids.

Step two. Remove all the goats to different accommodation, or pasture with shelters.

Step three. Muck-out the goathouse, clean and disinfect, leave empty for as long as possible but a minimum of two weeks. This allows any lice or eggs in the goathouse to die off or hatch and die off.
Step four. Re-apply the treatment, after a two week interval, to all the goats in their new (temporary) accommodation.

Step five. Wait a few days to allow any remaining lice to be killed by the second application of insecticide and the goats can then return to the original goathouse. Ideally the goathouse should be rested for a month.

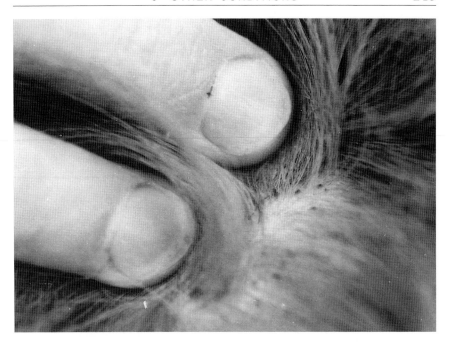

PLATE 8.13   Lice in the coat

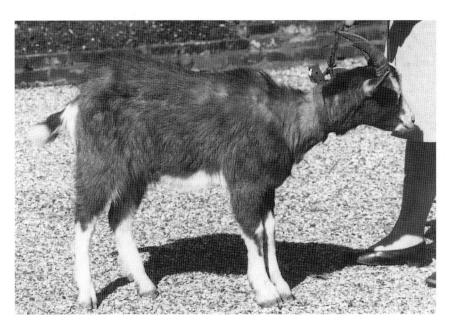

PLATE 8.14   Lice infestation – general appearance

If one does achieve eradication of the lice from the herd then care must be taken to quarantine incoming goats before they join the herd. (*See* page 13, Herd Management Policy.)

The parasiticides for the control of lice
In the UK no parasiticdes are licensed. In the USA, permethrin (a pyrethroid) is licensed and is widely used. There are some pour-on permethrin products licensed for use in cattle available in the UK. Cypermethrin is effective, used in the same way. To be used when the goats are not lactating. Wear protective rubber gloves when handling these preparations.

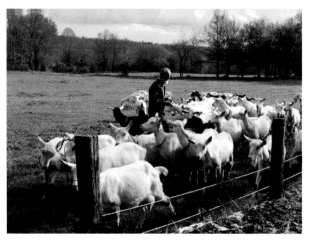

PLATE 8.15   Inspect grazing stock frequently.

HARVEST MITE INFESTATION

Infestation with this mite causes irritation and rubbing. It is mainly seen as greasy areas on the legs and lower body. The infestation commences in early autumn. The mites are red and can be seen with the aid of a magnifying glass.

Treatment
If possible, the goats should be moved to a different pasture. These mites do not normally pose a serious problem and treatment is not usually necessary, the problem tends to resolve as cooler weather approaches. Owners may find themselves with skin irritations caused by the same mites!

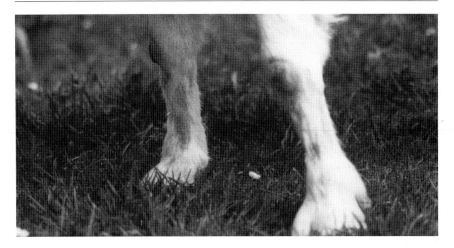

PLATE 8.16   Harvest mite infestation

WARTS AND PAPILLOMAS

These are most commonly found on the udder and teats, but they can occur anywhere. American workers have observed that warts found on the udder region fall into four categories:

- Those that disappear
- Those that reoccur in the summer
- Those that remain all year
- Those that become cancerous.

There are several factors which are relevant to the occurrence of warts, and they include exposure to sunlight, the absence of pigment in the skin, the age of the goat and possibly infective agents. It is believed that goats with unpigmented skin exposed to long hours of sunlight develop warts more commonly than goats with pigmented skin.

Treatment
Because the cause of the warts is in question the treatment is not always easy. They can be a nuisance at milking when on the teat. Many warts disappear with time, probably due to the development of viral immunity. Some may be easily removed by tying cotton thread around the base of them in order to cut off the blood supply. This can only be done with warts that have a 'stalk'. Discuss this with your vet.

SOME HEALTH ASPECTS OF FIBRE GOATS (ANGORA, CASHMERE ETC.)

Whilst the main emphasis of this book is upon the dairy goat, most subjects apply equally to the hair producing goats. There are a few special topics of importance to stress about the health and husbandry of the hair (or fibre) goats. The first subject to mention is hair. The goats we are discussing produce mainly soft undercoat as opposed to coarser guard hairs and undercoat.

NUTRITION

The most important topic to stress is that of adequate feeding, because the growth of hair requires lots of protein in the diet. If adequate protein is not supplied, then the goat continues to produce the hair at the expense of her other bodily functions, be it pregnancy, lactation or growth. Thus the fibre goat's diet has to be compared with that of the dairy goat during lactation. Two important points to bear in mind are: firstly, that Angora goats receiving inadequate feeding produce a greater quantity of large diameter fibre (undesirable). Secondly, if feeding in pregnancy is insufficient, then the effects are seen in the hair growth of the kid in utero. Thus kids with poor coats may result from poor feeding of the mother one year previously. Intimately tied up with nutrition is, of course, the mineral intake. This must be adequate, especially in relation to sulphur. Mohair contains high proportions of sulphur, containing amino-acids cystine and methionine. In order to supplement this, ammonium sulphate or sodium sulphate may be fed.

ABORTIONS

Most information on fibre goats comes from the United States and South Africa where large numbers of Angora goats are reared. Two forms of abortion are frequently reported.

Habitual Abortion
This is described in reports from South Africa and it can affect many animals in a herd. The aborted kid is found dead and is typically swollen. This form of abortion is not associated with

any infectious agents. In order to avoid the problem, the aborters are culled and only well grown, strong females kept for mating.

Stress Abortion
This has been seen in the USA; mainly young, underfed does abort, between 90 and 120 days gestation. The cause is considered to be a diet with insufficient 'energy' food in it (low in carbohydrate). The chain of events that result in the abortion are thought to be the following: low blood sugar levels in the mother and foetus cause the release of oestrogens (via the kid's adrenal glands). The oestrogens then act upon the uterus to stimulate the abortion. It is interesting to note that the foetuses are often produced alive.

REPRODUCTION AND FERTILITY

There is much written on this subject about the situation in the United States, where kidding rates for Angoras are often poor. (Kidding rate is the percentage of kids born per 100 does.) In the USA small females release poor numbers of eggs and hence very few kids. Essentially it's all back to nutrition. It must be remembered that the USA ranch conditions are much more severe than those experienced by the average Angora in the UK. Kid losses can be minimised, as with all goats, by paying attention to the provision of shelter at kidding time.

PARASITES

Worm Parasites
The Angora is particularly susceptible to the *Haemonchus* worm (a blood sucker). A heavy challenge results in anaemia of the goat and poorer coat quality. To check for anaemia see Plate 5.2 on page 108.

In the USA, *Parelaphostrongylus tenuis*, which is a parasite of the white tailed deer, can cause paralysis of the goat. This occurs when the worms migrate through the spinal cord. (For treatment for internal parasites *see* Chapter 5, page 85).

External Parasites
Probably the most important parasite in the UK is the biting

louse, *Damalinia caprae*. Obviously any parasite that causes the goats to rub and scratch themselves, causes damage to the valuable hair coat. Inspection of fleeces has to be a priority all the year round, though especially in the winter (the most active time for lice). The optimum time for treatment is 4 to 5 weeks after shearing when there is some regrowth to take up the chemical. The selection of insecticides available is wider for hair goats than for dairy goats. (There is no milk-withdrawal time to consider.) Fenvalerate, malathion, coumaphos or permethrines can be used. Care must be taken by the humans handling any of these compounds.

COCCIDIOSIS

This is apt to occur in situations where range goats are brought together for shearing. If weather conditions are bad there is a tendency to house the goats to prevent hypothermia. This often means that goats with weak immunity are collected together and come into contact with a heavy challenge from coccidia at a time when they are already stressed. (*See* page 67.)

Chapter 9

ACCIDENTS, EMERGENCIES AND POISONING

ACCIDENTS, EMERGENCIES AND FIRST AID

These types of problems fall into two categories, firstly those that the goatkeeper can treat and secondly those for which first-aid treatment should be given before your veterinary surgeon arrives. If in doubt, carry out the first aid and then ring your vet for his opinion as to what needs to be done. For quick reference, I shall list the topics that I shall cover in this chapter.

- Control of bleeding
- Tear wounds (lacerations)
- Stab wounds
- Choke
- Bloat
- Electric shock
- Snake bite
- Fractures
- Objects in the eye
- Sick goats

CONTROL OF BLEEDING

How to manage this problem depends upon where it is on the goat. If the bleeding is somewhere on a limb it is easier to deal with than bleeding from other places because a tourniquet can be applied for a short time. If the bleeding is severe, then although one should be as hygienic as possible, the immediate danger to the animal is loss of blood. In these instances, the first-aider is obliged to plunge in and do something quickly.

Arresting Bleeding from a Limb

For a tourniquet, a piece of stick and a length of string or baling twine are required. The twine is looped around the leg and wound over the stick so that the stick acts as a lever tightening the twine when turned. The tourniquet is applied between the body and the wound, for example in plate 9.1 the tourniquet would function for any wound on the lower part of the limb.

Never leave the tourniquet on for long, otherwise irreversible damage can result. In a case of severe bleeding apply a tourniquet, then ring your vet; return and release the tourniquet from time to time (every fifteen minutes) until he arrives. If the haemorrhage is not very severe, clean the wound with cotton wool

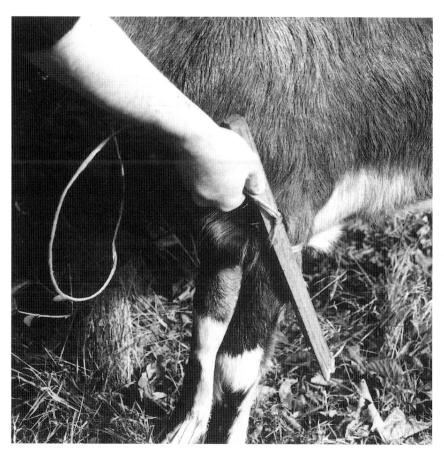

PLATE 9.1   Applying a tourniquet using baling twine and a stick

soaked in dilute antiseptic (e.g. Dettol), clip the hair all round the wound, bathe the wound again and then apply a dressing. The dressing consists of bandage or clean (old) cotton sheets. If you have an antiseptic dusting powder, apply that before bandaging. Finally, release the tourniquet.

Control of Bleeding from Elsewhere

This is more difficult and the principle is to apply direct pressure using a clean material such as an old cotton sheet. If severe, your veterinary surgeon will have to deal with it, probably by stitching. A small wound may be temporarily plugged with a piece of gauze.

TEAR WOUNDS OR LACERATIONS

If the bleeding is not severe then these may be treated by the owner provided that the goat has been vaccinated against tetanus. Clean up the area with cold water and clip away hairs from the edge of the wound. Use tweezers to remove any foreign bodies such as splinters of wood. Irrigate the wound with dilute antiseptic such as Dettol. Allow it to dry and then apply antiseptic powder. Smear Vaseline around the wound and apply a clean dressing of gauze and bandage.

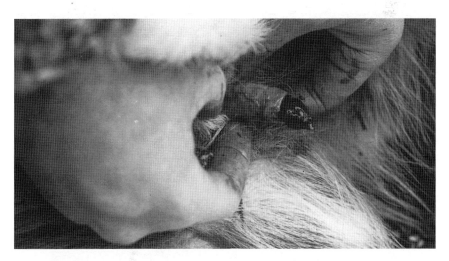

PLATE 9.2   Bleeding from penis resulting from attempting to leap over a barrier

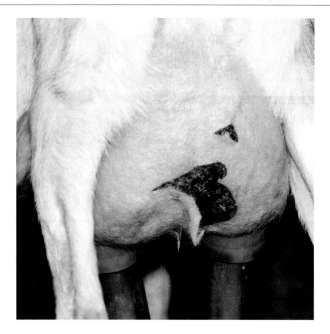

PLATE 9.3 & 9.4   Tear wounds: before suturing and 2 days afterwards.
(NB: Large wounds are often less serious than puncture wounds)

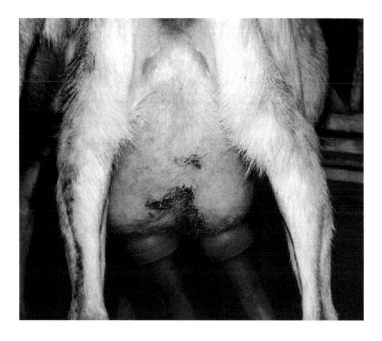

In hot weather a fly-repellent should be used, preferably one combined with antiseptic powder.

STAB WOUNDS

Wounds that result from a spike or similar object penetrating the skin and muscles are potentially very dangerous. Do not be lulled into a false sense of security by the small size of the hole. The reason, of course, is that any infection that may have entered tends to become trapped inside. It cannot be washed and cleaned from the outside and thus one normally has to rely on antibiotic injections. Tetanus is the most serious result of this type of wound, if any of your goats suffer such an accident obtain professional help quickly.

CHOKE

Obstruction of the oesophagus (gullet) in the ruminant is of much more consequence than a similar problem in, say, a human. The reason of course is that gas is constantly being produced in the rumen and it has to get out, otherwise the rumen fills up like a balloon (bloat).

Pieces of apple or carrot, for example, may lodge in the oesophagus. Sometimes the bulge can be seen or felt on the left-hand side of the neck near the windpipe. If possible, try and milk the object down into the stomach by applying massage to the neck.

If this fails, let your veterinary surgeon deal with it. Should the goat be in a very distressed state, puncture the rumen (see BLOAT, following).

BLOAT EMERGENCY TREATMENT

Only carry out the following if the goat is in danger of death; otherwise refer to BLOAT, page 139.

Take a very sharp knife and stab the left-hand flank in the area indicated in plate 9.5. When a goat is bloated the area which can be stabbed is quite large. It will be fairly obvious because it is soft when pressed. Put the knife in well behind the rib cage and fairly high up, because the gas will be at the top of the rumen. A fairly 'high' stab prevents leakage of rumen contents into the peritoneum.

It is not an easy thing to do, because the stomach behaves as if it were a balloon. Remove the knife and the gas will escape rapidly.

After this emergency action, consult your vet, as the underlying problem may persist and it may be necessary to give the goat antibiotic treatment.

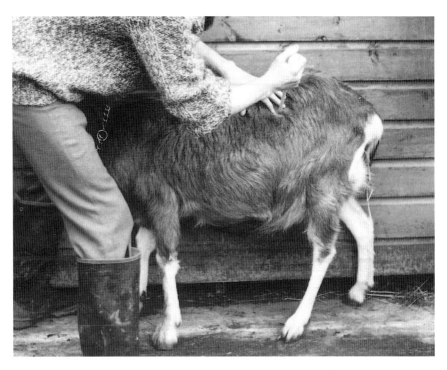

PLATE 9.5   Correct site for the emergency relief of bloat

ELECTRIC SHOCK

Switch off the current before touching the goat! If you think that she is still alive stimulate her by massage. Keep her warm using plenty of straw or a rug over her back.

Prevention
Keep all electrical fittings high, out of the range of goats. Remember that goats can reach up to two metres!

Snake Bites

Occasionally to be found in goats, snake bites are generally seen at the front end, particularly the lips, muzzle and neck. Swelling is noted; the goat may appear shocked and two fang marks may be detected. The swelling is very painful and causes concern to the goat.

Treatment
It is probably wise to get your veterinary surgeon to examine the bitten goat because the effects can be fatal. If the bite is on the leg, then the application of a tourniquet is advisable (for a short period) in an attempt to localise the toxin. Antibiotics are useful because many of the bites are infected with germs of tetanus and gangrene. Specific antiserum is available for injection into the goat should the emergency arise.

Fractures

I have only seen fractures of the forelegs, usually those are of kids, trapped between horizontal bars. Active kids may attempt to jump from one pen into another and in doing so, sometimes catch their legs. Pen walls should always be sufficiently high to prevent this occurring.

First aid
Leave the goat quiet and summon your veterinary surgeon. You could attempt a rough splint as a temporary measure, but most animals with fractures will lie quiet and still. An adult goat should be propped on her brisket with bales in order to avoid bloat developing. It may be necessary for someone to stay with the goat in order to give her support.

Treatment
This very much depends upon where the fracture is; those below the knee or hock can be treated by external support, splint or plaster cast. Breaks high up on the leg may only be repaired by surgical technique and the goat would have to be extremely valuable to warrant the expense.

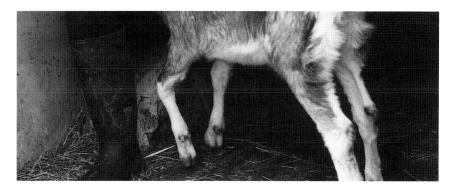

PLATE 9.6   Fracture below the knee

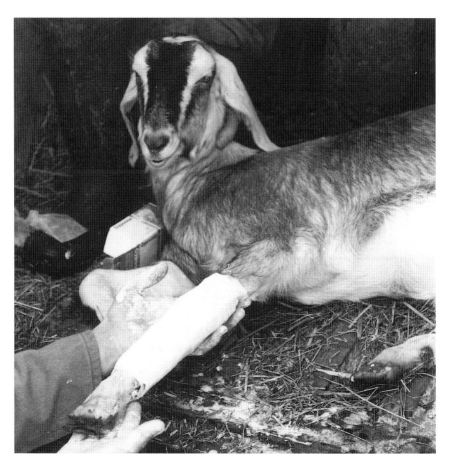

PLATE 9.7   Applying the plaster cast

COLIC

The pain that results from digestive upsets can be very severe and the goat will appear very distressed. Fortunately the pain is generally spasmodic and will pass off fairly quickly. Keeping the goat occupied by walking her will normally be enough treatment until the pain passes. If the problem persists your veterinary surgeon will probably give the goat a smooth muscle relaxant drug such as Buscopan (Boehringer Ingelheim).

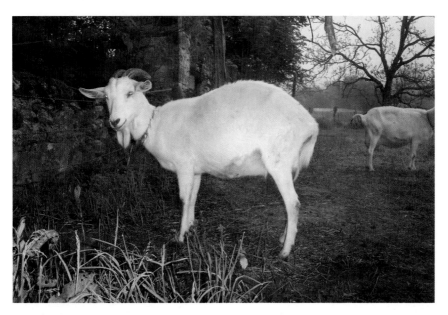

PLATE 9.8   Colic – arched back and vocalising

FOREIGN BODY IN THE EYE

A hay seed may fall into the goat's eye and require to be removed. If it cannot be readily pulled from the eye, use a little sugar to stimulate tears; dissolve a little sugar and drop it into the eye. Failing this, touch the object lightly with a greased brush to pick it out.

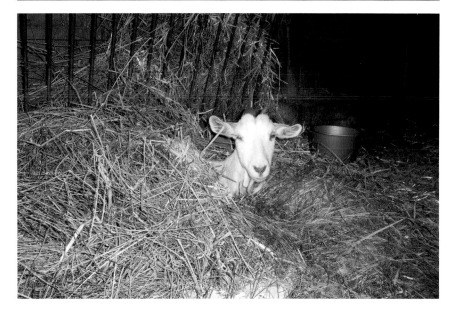

PLATE 9.9   Nursing care – sick goat

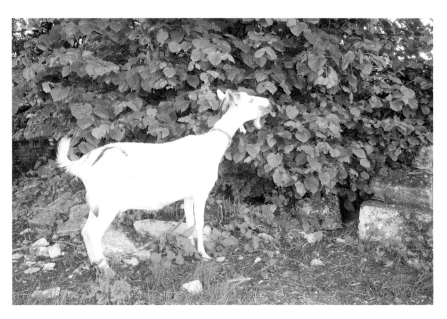

PLATE 9.10   Recovered Goat – after 48 hours (the same goat as
              Plates 9.8 and 9.9)

Treatment of any Sick Goat

Any sick goat will always benefit from a drink of tepid water especially if it contains a teaspoonful of common salt to each litre.

POISONING

Lead Poisoning

There are very few reports of lead poisoning in goats, although there are several descriptions of experimental poisoning.

Lead is fairly commonly found around farms and homes, being present in paint, putty, batteries and felt. Goats are less inclined to lick lead objects but they may chew at wood and take in lead from paint at the same time.

Symptoms
The layman will be unable to distinguish the symptoms from those of many other diseases such as CCN (*see* page 91). Blindness, incoordination, head-pressing and teeth-grinding are all seen.

Treatment
Some goats will respond to treatment but many will be too far gone and die. Injections of a substance known as calcium versenate will be given by your veterinary surgeon into the goat's vein. Drenching the goat with magnesium sulphate will help prevent the further absorption of lead from the intestine. The goatkeeper could drench the goat with two teaspoonfuls of Epsom salts dissolved in water while waiting for the veterinary surgeon to arrive. This action can still be taken even if you are not sure it is lead poisoning – it won't do any harm. Because the symptoms are identical to several other diseases showing similar nervous symptoms, laboratory tests may have to be carried out. From a live animal, a blood sample will be collected, but if one animal from a group has died, then the kidneys will be collected from it at post-mortem examination. The kidneys will be used for laboratory testing.

Prevention
Always try to prevent goats coming into contact with sources of lead, especially lead paint.

Public health precautions
Heavy metals such as lead are of course poisonous to humans. Advice should be sought as to whether the carcase would be fit for human consumption, following such a diagnosis. Some countries, including the UK, impose restrictions on the animals involved until they are deemed fit for human consumption.

FLUORIDE POISONING

See FLUOROSIS, page 127.

PENTACHLOROPHENOL POISONING

Goats can succumb to poisoning with this substance, used abundantly as a timber preservative. Do not allow goats access to timber treated in this way until it is thoroughly dry.

Symptoms
Convulsions and other nervous symptoms followed by death.

Treatment
There is no specific antidote and the prospect is extremely poor. Your veterinary surgeon may try using non-specific treatment but there is nothing that will help much.

DIESEL FUEL POISONING

Poisoning with this substance is reported to give rise to dullness, pneumonia and nervous symptoms. As with many poisons there is no specific antidote but supportive therapy with fluids and vitamins may help.

NITRATE (NITRITE) POISONING

Symptoms of nitrate poisoning are excitement, staggering, prostration, muscle tremor, increased respiration, frothing at the mouth and death. This may occur in goats grazing pasture that has recently had artificial fertilizer applied to it. Generally, the nitrate is broken down to nitrite in the rumen. Treatment is not very successful. Methylene blue (2 per cent solution) can be injected intravenously. Oily substances by mouth may help to protect the intestines from irritation.

PLANT POISONING

There are a tremendous range of plants that can poison goats, many of them giving rise to a wide range of symptoms. In my experience, only a limited number of them are commonly seen and these I shall cover in detail. It is outside the scope of this book to deal with all the other possible causes of poisoning and the reader could refer to the HMSO publication number 161 *Poisonous Plants in Britain* for further information. Some general comments about plant poisoning in goats are worthwhile noting.

The Quantity of Plant Eaten
If only small quantities of dangerous plants are eaten, then the effects may be very slight. This is especially true if the goat has a rumen full of 'safe' food such as hay or grass. In this case the poison is 'diluted' in the rumen and has less effect.

The Husbandry System
When given a choice, goats on extensive grazing or browse tend to avoid poisonous plants. This is true of course until food becomes scarce in which case the goats may be forced to eat poisonous plants. If goats which are accustomed to being yarded are given the rare chance to browse they may take the opportunity to try anything within their reach and perhaps poison themselves.

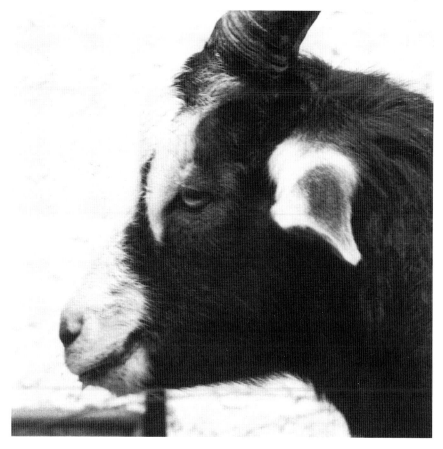

PLATE 9.11   Goat suffering from rhododendron poisoning

Rhododendron Poisoning

This is the most common type of poisoning that I see: even a few leaves seem to cause the symptoms to develop. The toxin involved is andromedotoxin.

Symptoms
Characteristically, the goats retch, vomit, salivate and become very depressed. Sometimes they are ill for several days and develop laboured breathing.

Treatment
Ephedrine may be given at a dose rate of 1 mg/kg of body weight, in order to counteract the effect of the toxin upon the heart. Vitamin injections are very useful in order to speed up the detoxification of the poison. If your goat is not vaccinated against enterotoxaemia your vet will probably prescribe a penicillin injection because of the poison's effect on the digestive system. If the goat is valuable, your vet may perform an operation to remove all the stomach contents, via the left flank.

Drenching with tea may be attempted whilst you are waiting for the veterinary surgeon. Drenching is not recommended if the goat is still retching badly because the fluids may enter the windpipe and go into the lungs.

Many affected goats will pull through if well nursed, although the poisoning can be fatal.

RAGWORT POISONING

Ragwort is common in the United Kingdom and causes severe damage to the liver. It grows in many parts of the world including the USA and New Zealand. The damage is gradual and irreversible, so there is no treatment for affected animals. The symptoms reflect the damage to the liver and include loss of condition, poor appetite and anaemia. In very severe cases the eyes and mouth become yellow due to the development of jaundice. Hay containing dried ragwort is still dangerous to animals.

KALE POISONING

Kale or rape is frequently fed to cattle and sometimes to goats. Excessive quantities can result in damage to the red blood cells which rupture. This results in the breakdown products of blood being lost in the urine. One of the symptoms of poisoning is, therefore, red urine. Other symptoms which may follow are weakness and anaemia. If kale poisoning develops, the only treatment normally required is to move the goats off the kale and on to other forages such as grass or hay.

OXALATE POISONING

Plants such as sugar beet tops or rhubarb can give rise to symptoms of hypocalcaemia (*see* MILK FEVER page 143). Treatment involves the administration of calcium borogluconate in order to reverse this state.

OAK LEAF POISONING

Excessive feeding of oak leaves may lead to damage to the bone marrow and subsequently anaemia. The bone marrow is essential for producing red blood cells and if it is damaged fewer red blood cells are manufactured, which leads to anaemia. Oak leaves fed in moderation are fairly harmless.

FRUIT TREE LEAF POISONING (PRUNUS)
(Plums and Cherries)

The leaves of the prunus family are poisonous to goats because they contain a cyanogenetic glycoside called amygdalin. When fresh, the leaves are harmless but when dry and wilted they contain hydrogen cyanide. This compound combines with the oxygen-carrying structure of the red blood cell making it unable to carry oxygen. The symptoms are those of lack of oxygen with bright cherry red colour to the mouth and other membranes. Treatment involves the administration of sodium nitrite and sodium thiosulphate into the vein. Substances to stimulate breathing would help but the course of the disease may be too rapid for treatment to be given.

APPENDICES

REFERENCES

JOURNALS

Advances in Sheep and Goat Medicine.
Veterinary Clinics of North America, Food Animal Practice, Vol. 6.,
  No. 3, Nov. 1990, 'Special Problems of Hair Goats'.
British Goat Society Journal.
Dairy Goat Journal, Scottsdale, Arizona, U.S.A.
Farmers Weekly, London.
Goat Veterinary Society Journal, BVA, London.
International Sheep and Goat Research, Scottsdale, Arizona, U.S.A.
Journal of the American Veterinary Medical Association.
Symposium of the American Sheep and Goat Practitioners (1976).
The Veterinary Record, BVA, London.
La Chèvre, 149, rue de Bercy, 75595. Paris cedex 12.
Les Maladies nerveuses du Mouton et de la Chèvre. Supplement
  technique. No. 32 à la Dépêche Veterinaire. 15–21 Mai 1993.
Also world-wide selection of journals and abstracts.

BOOKS

Blood, D.C and Radostits, O.M. (1990), *Veterinary Medicine*,
  Baillière 7th Edn., London.
British Poisonous Plants and Fungi (1988), HMSO, London,
  Bulletin 161.
Duphar Vitamin Guide for Feedmen and Veterinarians, Duphar,
  Amsterdam.
Gall, C. (1981, 1985), *Goat Production*, Academic Press, London.
Guss, S.B. (1977), *Management and Diseases of Dairy Goats*, Dairy
  Goat Publishing Corporation, Scottsdale, Arizona 85252.
Hetherington, L. (1979), *All About Goats*, 3rd Edn., Farming Press,
  Ipswich.

271

Mackenzie, D. (1993), *Goat Husbandry*, 5th Edn., Faber, London.
Matthews, J. (1991), *Outline of Clinical Diagnosis in the Goat*, Wright.
Merck Veterinary Annual (1991), 7th Edn., Merck and Co., Rahway, N.J., U.S.A.
Mowlem Alan (1988), *Goat Farming*, 2nd Edn., Farming Press, Ipswich.
Thiel, C. C. and Dodd, F. H. (editors) (1992), *Machine Milking and Lactation*, N.I.R.D., Reading.
Abbott, K.A., Taylor, M., Stubbings, L.A., Sustainable worm control strategies for sheep, SCOPS, UK.
Various authors (2004), *Guide sanitaire de l'elevage caprin*. FRGDS, Poitou-Charentes.
Defra (2004), *Guidance on control of Johne's disease in dairy herds*, PB9990.
NOAH (2005), *Compendium of animal medicines, Enfield*.

WEBSITES
Defra. www.defra.gov.uk
Also world-wide selection.

GOAT PHYSIOLOGICAL DATA

Great care should be taken in interpreting the following 'normal' measurements because they are extremely variable. These measurements should be taken when the goat is rested. It is no use counting the goat's breathing, for example, after chasing it round a field. The body temperature should be interpreted after comparing the temperature of two other animals in the group.

Body temperature	38.5–40°C
Pulse	77–89 beats per minute
Breathing rate	15–25 per minute
Age at puberty	4–5 months (male and female)
Season	September to February (approx.) in northern hemisphere. March to August in southern hemisphere
Duration of oestrus (heat)	12–48 hours
Length between heats	19–21 days (within the season)
Pregnancy	146–154 days (average 150)
Weight	Adult female 55–100 kg
	Adult male 75–110 kg

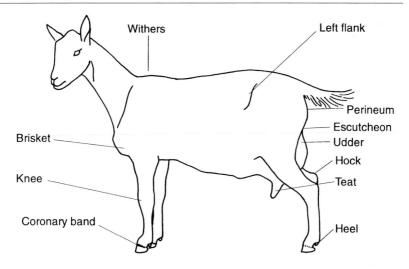

Points of the goat

INFORMATION FROM A GVS GOAT HEALTH SURVEY*

Approximately 1,000 goats in 69 herds were surveyed over the course of a year. Owners or their veterinary surgeon completed an incident form whenever anything happened to the goat. What follows is some of the information gained.

STATISTICS

227 incidents were reported, the outcomes of which were as follows:

	Number	As a percentage of incidents	As a percentage of goats
Recovered	194	85.46	Not relevant
Died	15	6.60	1.5
Euthanased	11	4.84	1.1
Culled	7	3.08	0.7

* This information comes by courtesy of the Goat Veterinary Society and was collected and processed by the author. Thanks to the co-operating goatkeepers and veterinary surgeons and to my neighbour Mr Robin Swale for his help in processing the data.

COMMENTS

Even if the 'died' and 'euthanased' categories are combined, mortality in goats, as indicated by this survey, is very low compared with other farm species.

Similarly the culling of poor and unproductive goats is extremely low. This may reflect the sentimental attachment of some owners to their goats. Goats are possibly kept longer than straight financial considerations would dictate.

The Anglo-Nubian breed records a strikingly high number of problems. There was not a significantly predominant group of them in this survey, and they were kept in only 18 herds.

Tables 1 and 2 follow on pages 275 and 276.

PROBLEMS ENCOUNTERED

Alimentary (Digestive) Problems
As can be seen from Table 1, the most commonly encountered problems affected the alimentary (digestive) system, and these were predominantly associated with diarrhoea. Bloat was encountered in 4 goats and was fatal in 1 kid.

Skin problems
These were the second most commonly reported group. Manges, especially chorioptic mange, predominated. Chorioptic mange was largely reported in the winter.

Reproductive problems
Difficult kiddings were the most numerous problems in this group, with Anglo-Nubians forming the single most-reported breed.

Udder disease
Mastitis was diagnosed on 12 occasions; it was recorded in most breeds and took up to 21 days to clear in one goat. The other problems were mainly cuts and sores.

Locomotor system
There was no predominant problem in this category, which included foot sepsis, arthritis, splinters and a fracture.

Metabolic problems

Ketosis (acetonaemia) was the predominant finding in this category, emphasising the importance of this problem after kidding. Hypocalcamia was recorded only twice and hypogagnesaemia once. The poisonings were all due to rhododendrons.

Respiratory disease

This affected young and old alike and was surprisingly more a feature of the non-winter months, being absent from November to February. No fatal cases were reported.

Off-colour

This category recorded goats with few specific symptoms that recovered with or without treatment in 1 to 5 days. The majority were lactating females.

Nervous conditions

There were few specific diagnoses in this category except for lead poisoning in 1 kid. Half the cases died or were put to sleep.

TABLE 1—BREEDS AND THE CONDITIONS AFFECTING THEM

DIAGNOSIS

	AL	CO	DEP	EY	LOC	MET	NER	OFF	PU	PYR	REP	RES	SK	UDD	UR	ALL
Not stated	0	0	0	0	0	0	0	0	0	0	0	0	1	1	0	2
ALP	4	0	0	0	2	0	0	0	0	0	1	1	1	3	1	13
ALPX	0	0	0	0	0	0	0	0	0	0	0	0	1	0	0	1
ANG	2	0	0	0	0	0	0	0	0	0	0	0.	0	0	0	2
ANGx	0	0	0	0	0	0	0	0	0	0	0	0	0	0	1	1
BRI	3	0	0	0	1	2	1	1	0	1	2	0	6	1	0	18
BRIX	0	0	0	0	0	0	0	1	0	0	0	0	0	0	0	1
CX	0	0	0	0	0	0	0	0	0	0	0	0	0	0	1	1
ENG	4	1	0	0	0	2	0	0	2	0	2	0	3	2	0	16
ENGX	0	0	0	0	0	1	0	0	0	0	0	0	0	0	0	1
GG	5	0	0	0	1	1	3	0	0	0	0	0	0	1	0	11
NUB	20	1	0	2	8	4	1	6	1	0	14	5	13	5	0	80
NUBX	0	0	0	0	0	1	0	0	0	0	0	0	0	0	0	1
SAA	7	0	2	1	4	5	0	2	0	3	2	3	5	4	0	38
SAAX	0	0	0	0	1	0	1	0	0	0	0	0	1	0	1	4
TOG	8	0	0	0	2	1	0	1	0	0	5	3	14	3	0	37
Total	53	2	2	3	19	17	6	11	3	4	26	12	45	20	4	227

Key to abbreviations on page 276

TABLE 2—THE MONTH OF INCIDENCE, MAY 1983–MAY 1984

	Month not stated	1	2	3	4	5	6	7	8	9	10	11	12	ALL
AL	0	0	1	3	5	7	6	10	3	6	2	7	3	53
CO	0	0	0	0	1	0	0	1	0	0	0	0	0	2
DEP	0	0	0	0	0	0	0	0	0	0	1	1	0	2
EY	0	0	1	0	0	2	0	0	0	0	0	0	0	3
LOC	0	2	2	1	1	2	0	2	0	4	0	4	1	19
MET	0	0	1	4	0	3	1	0	1	0	4	1	2	17
NER	0	0	0	1	1	0	1	0	0	2	0	1	0	6
OFF	0	1	0	0	0	3	2	0	2	0	1	2	0	11
PU	2	0	0	1	0	0	0	0	0	0	0	0	0	3
PYR	0	0	0	0	0	0	2	2	0	0	0	0	0	4
REP	0	3	3	6	4	3	1	0	0	0	0	3	3	26
RES	0	0	0	2	1	3	2	1	1	1	1	0	0	12
SK	1	5	3	2	6	7	6	4	2	2	1	1	5	45
UDD	1	0	1	1	2	4	5	1	0	0	2	3	0	20
UR	0	1	0	0	0	3	0	0	0	0	0	0	0	4
Total	4	12	12	21	21	37	26	21	9	15	12	23	14	227

Key to Abbreviations

DIAGNOSIS

AL: alimentary (digestive system)
CO: collapsed
DEP: depressed milk yield
EY: eye
LOC: locomotor (muscles and joints)
MET: metabolic
NER: nervous
OFF: off-colour
PU: pyrexia (fever) of unknown origin
PYR: pyrexia
REP: reproductive
RES: respiratory (breathing system)
SK: skin (except udder)
UDD: udder (udder and teats)
UR:-urinary system (kidneys, bladder, etc.)

BREED

ALP: Alpine
ANG: Angora
BRI: British
CX: Cross-breed
GG: Golden Guernsey
NUB: Nubian
SAA: Saanen
TOG: Toggenburg ENG: English

X indicates cross of breed

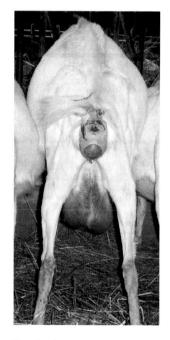

Replacing a prolapsed vagina is a fairly simple operation (*see* pp. 196–7)

INDEX

Note: page numbers in *italics* refer to figures and plates

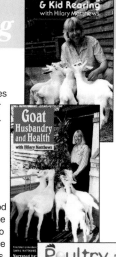
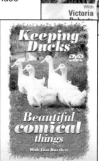
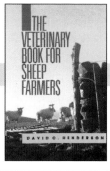